Cases for Nursing Simulation: A Student Guide

Jean Yockey, MSN, RN, FNP, CNE
University of South Dakota

Larinda Dixon, Ed.D, RN, MSN
College of DuPage

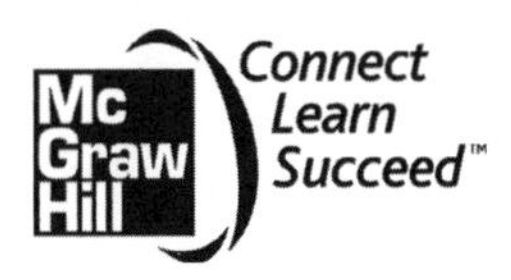

The McGraw·Hill Companies

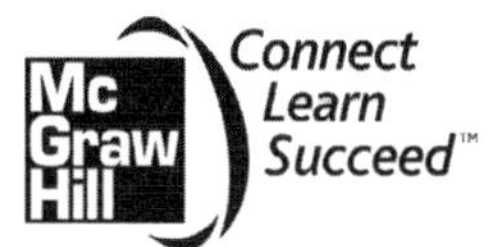

CASES FOR NURSING SIMULATION: A STUDENT GUIDE

Published by McGraw-Hill, a business unit of The McGraw-Hill Companies, Inc., 1221 Avenue of the Americas, New York, NY, 10020.

This book is printed on acid-free paper.

1 2 3 4 5 6 7 8 9 0 QDB/QDB 1 0 9 8 7 6 5 4 3 2 1

ISBN 978-0-07-340228-4

MHID 0-07-340228-1

Vice president/Editor in chief: *Elizabeth Haefele*
Vice president/Director of marketing: *Alice Harra*
Publisher: *Kenneth S. Kasee Jr.*
Managing developmental editor: *Kimberly D. Hooker*
Editorial coordinator: *Jenna Skwarek*
Marketing manager: *Mary B. Haran*
Lead digital product manager: *Damian Moshak*
Director, Editing/Design/Production: *Jess Ann Kosic*
Lead project manager: *Susan Trentacosti*
Buyer: *Nicole Baumgartner*
Senior designer: *Srdjan Savanovic*
Digital production coordinator: *Brent dela Cruz*
Cover design: *Srdjan Savanovic*
Typeface: *CRC*
Compositor: *Laserwords Private Limited*
Printer: *Quad/Graphics*
Cover credit: *Area9*

www.mhhe.com

CONTENTS

READ ME FIRST!

INTRODUCTION

Welcome to the world of learning with simulation! Simulation allows you to learn and practice how to act and react in patient encounters. You can use simulation without being in clinical agencies. Having time to prepare, perform, and review allows for reflection on learning, and the experience to make appropriate care decisions when caring for real patients.

There are 10 simulation cases presented in this book. Featured characters are based on major concepts that nurses need to understand to provide safe care to patients in the health care environment. Each simulation allows the practice of nursing care as it relates to each concept. Patient safety and reaching desired care outcomes is dependent on the competence of the healthcare persons providing care. Building competence comes by building on previous knowledge and skills. It comes with practice in making quick and safe decisions, and gaining clinical experience. Treating the simulations as a real patient situation will help you transfer your learning to the clinical setting.

An important part of the learning process is preparing for patient care, and then applying this knowledge by caring for real patients. Simulation allows the learner to practice the application of knowledge in a setting that is safe, and with patient conditions that can change over time. Communication skills are improved as your team works together to coordinate and provide care for the patients.

How to Use the Simulation Scenarios

The simulations are divided into two sections. The first section gives background information on the clinical situation and how to prepare for the simulation.

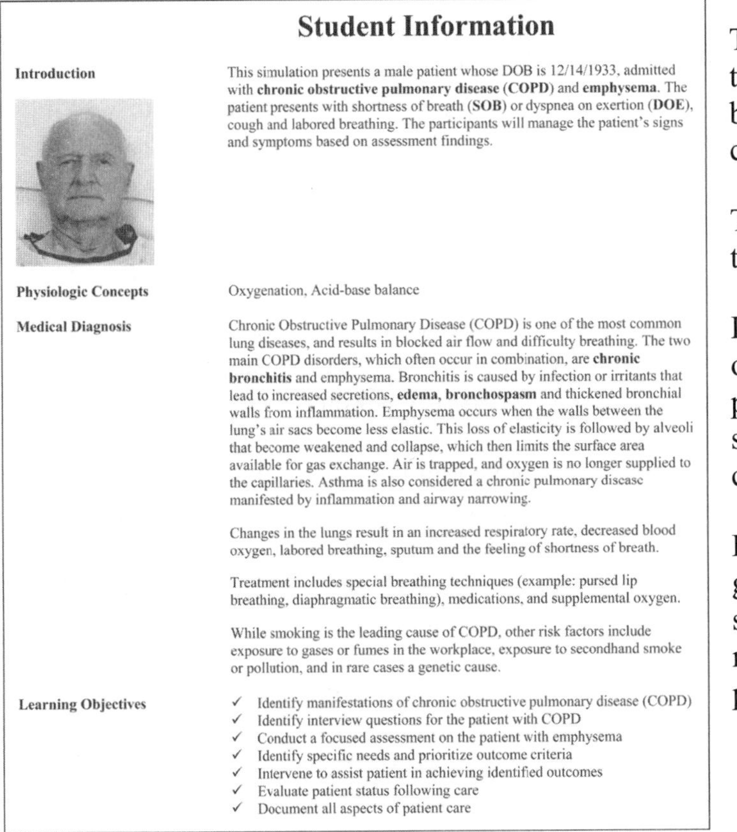

Student Information

Introduction	This simulation presents a male patient whose DOB is 12/14/1933, admitted with **chronic obstructive pulmonary disease (COPD)** and **emphysema**. The patient presents with shortness of breath (**SOB**) or dyspnea on exertion (**DOE**), cough and labored breathing. The participants will manage the patient's signs and symptoms based on assessment findings.
Physiologic Concepts	Oxygenation, Acid-base balance
Medical Diagnosis	Chronic Obstructive Pulmonary Disease (COPD) is one of the most common lung diseases, and results in blocked air flow and difficulty breathing. The two main COPD disorders, which often occur in combination, are **chronic bronchitis** and emphysema. Bronchitis is caused by infection or irritants that lead to increased secretions, **edema, bronchospasm** and thickened bronchial walls from inflammation. Emphysema occurs when the walls between the lung's air sacs become less elastic. This loss of elasticity is followed by alveoli that become weakened and collapse, which then limits the surface area available for gas exchange. Air is trapped, and oxygen is no longer supplied to the capillaries. Asthma is also considered a chronic pulmonary disease manifested by inflammation and airway narrowing. Changes in the lungs result in an increased respiratory rate, decreased blood oxygen, labored breathing, sputum and the feeling of shortness of breath. Treatment includes special breathing techniques (example: pursed lip breathing, diaphragmatic breathing), medications, and supplemental oxygen. While smoking is the leading cause of COPD, other risk factors include exposure to gases or fumes in the workplace, exposure to secondhand smoke or pollution, and in rare cases a genetic cause.
Learning Objectives	✓ Identify manifestations of chronic obstructive pulmonary disease (COPD) ✓ Identify interview questions for the patient with COPD ✓ Conduct a focused assessment on the patient with emphysema ✓ Identify specific needs and prioritize outcome criteria ✓ Intervene to assist patient in achieving identified outcomes ✓ Evaluate patient status following care ✓ Document all aspects of patient care

The left-hand column identifies each topic for the section. Each simulation begins with a brief overview of the clinical situation being presented.

The physiologic concepts presented in the simulation are identified.

In the medical diagnosis section, an overview of the illness process is presented, including pathophysiology, signs and symptoms, risk factors, and common treatments for the condition.

Learning objectives can serve as a guide when preparing for the simulation. They can also be used as a measure of knowledge needed to provide care.

Simulation Setting

Adult Patient Medical Unit

Participant Preparation

Knowledge Preparation:

- Review the pathophysiology and clinical manifestations of COPD
- Review assessment needed for a patient with COPD
- Review laboratory and diagnostic findings related to the respiratory status of a patient with COPD
- Review safe oxygen delivery methods

Skill Preparation:

- Assessment, with a focus on respiratory and cardiovascular systems
- Application of oxygen delivery systems
- Medication administration, including inhaled route

Evidence-Based Practice Recommendations

1. All individuals identified as having **dyspnea** related to chronic obstructive pulmonary disease (COPD) will be assessed appropriately, to include: vital signs, respiratory assessment, cardiovascular assessment, and level of consciousness.
2. Nurses will be able to implement appropriate nursing interventions for all levels of dyspnea including acute episodes of respiratory distress. Interventions include safe administration of prescribed medications by various routes, controlled oxygen therapy, breathing strategies to help gas exchange and secretion clearance, activity tolerance plan and nutrition plan.
3. Education for the patient with COPD should include smoking cessation strategies if needed, breathing techniques, meeting nutritional needs, and accurate use of medication and inhaler devices.
4. Health Promotion includes administering pneumococcal vaccine and annual influenza vaccination for individuals without contraindications.

Are You Ready?

1. What questions would you ask a patient to assess for breathing difficulty?
2. What would you expect a patient to look like who is short of breath?
3. How would you administer medications that help open narrowed airways?
4. What are your priority nursing actions for a patient with **hypoxia**?

Continue on to meet the patient!

The setting for the patient situation is identified.

Participant preparation gives information on knowledge and skills needed to prepare to complete the simulation. The topics are intended to be used with your Medical-surgical text and nursing skill resources.

Evidence-based recommendations identify practice guidelines recommendations of national professional organizations.

Finally, a section is presented with review questions to allow assessment on readiness to complete the simulation.

Patient Information

Name	**Medical Record Number**	**Birth Date**	**Allergies**
Henry Winston	101-33-986	12/14/1933	Sulfonamides
Height	**Weight**	**Gender**	**Attending Physician**
65 inches	185 lbs	Male	Dr. Han Lee

Past Medical History

Previously diagnosed with emphysema. History of **MI**, **HTN**, Left-sided **heart failure**, fractured ankle.

Initial Vital Signs

T 98.4°F, P 88, R 20, B/P 126/84, SpO_2 93% **RA** on admit, Pain 4/10 with cough

? **Clinical Competency**

1. What is your interpretation of the patient's vital signs?

Physician Orders

Oxygen to maximum 4 L/min to keep pulse oximetry ≥ 90%
Prednisolone 80 mg po q day
Aspirin 81 mg po daily
Atrovent (ipratropium bromide) 2 puffs t.i.d.
Albuterol MDI 2 puffs q 6 hr prn
Lasix (furosemide) 40 mg po daily
Lopressor (metoprolol) 50 mg po bid
Lanoxin (digoxin) 0.125 mg po daily
CXR, CBC, Chem 7, Chem 15, ABGs, UA
Low sodium (4 gram) diet
Up with assistance
VS q 4 hours and prn
Saline lock
I/O

? **Clinical Competency**

2. Why is each medication prescribed for this patient?
3. Is each medication safe to administer to this patient?
4. What are concerns the nurse has with administering oxygen at a high flow rate to this patient?

Nurse Report

Henry Winston is a married male whose DOB is 12/14/1933, admitted after midnight with acute exacerbation of COPD. Assessment reveals an anxious man who is becoming more dyspneic with exertion. The **UAP** just got a pulse oximetry of 88% on RA. He does not use oxygen at home. Heart rate is regular. Respirations are labored, with right lower lobe crackles and wheezing bilaterally. He is up with assist but he is voiding per urinal as he does not tolerate getting up to the bathroom. Saline lock in place and patent.

The second section introduces you to the specific patient you will be caring for. This section begins with patient information. The physician orders are identified, allowing an opportunity to prepare for any unfamiliar terms or treatments.

The nurse report is in this section, and simulates the information that would be received from one nurse to another.

Note that there are clinical competency questions that ask for your interpretation and understanding of the clinical situation. Answers for these questions are found in Appendix A.

Continue on to the simulation section!

Cases for Nursing Simulation

Chronic Obstructive Pulmonary Disease
Student Information

Introduction

This simulation presents a male patient whose DOB is 12/14/1933, admitted with **chronic obstructive pulmonary disease** (**COPD**) and **emphysema**. The patient presents with shortness of breath (**SOB**) or dyspnea on exertion (**DOE**), cough and labored breathing. The participants will manage the patient's signs and symptoms based on assessment findings.

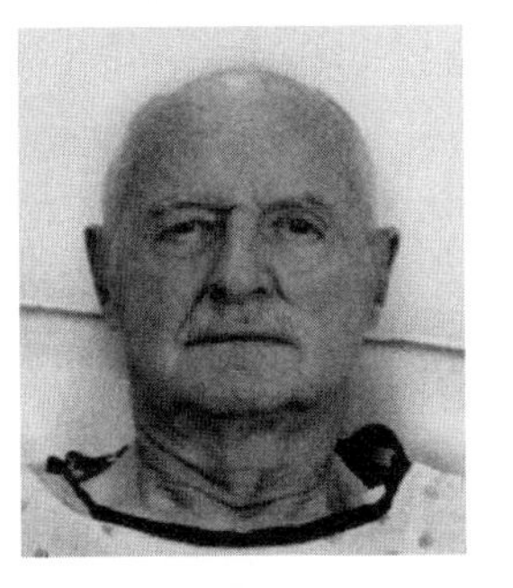

Physiologic Concepts

Oxygenation, Acid-base balance

Medical Diagnosis

Chronic Obstructive Pulmonary Disease (COPD) is one of the most common lung diseases, and results in blocked air flow and difficulty breathing. The two main COPD disorders, which often occur in combination, are **chronic bronchitis** and emphysema. Bronchitis is caused by infection or irritants that lead to increased secretions, **edema**, **bronchospasm** and thickened bronchial walls from inflammation. Emphysema occurs when the walls between the lung's air sacs become less elastic. This loss of elasticity is followed by alveoli that become weakened and collapse, which then limits the surface area available for gas exchange. Air is trapped, and oxygen is no longer supplied to the capillaries. Asthma is also considered a chronic pulmonary disease manifested by inflammation and airway narrowing.

Changes in the lungs result in an increased respiratory rate, decreased blood oxygen, labored breathing, sputum and the feeling of shortness of breath.

Treatment includes special breathing techniques (example: pursed lip breathing, diaphragmatic breathing), medications, and supplemental oxygen.

While smoking is the leading cause of COPD, other risk factors include exposure to gases or fumes in the workplace, exposure to secondhand smoke or pollution, and in rare cases a genetic cause.

Learning Objectives

- ✓ Identify manifestations of chronic obstructive pulmonary disease (COPD)
- ✓ Identify interview questions for the patient with COPD
- ✓ Conduct a focused assessment on the patient with emphysema
- ✓ Identify specific needs and prioritize outcome criteria
- ✓ Intervene to assist patient in achieving identified outcomes
- ✓ Evaluate patient status following care
- ✓ Document all aspects of patient care

Simulation Setting

Adult Patient Medical Unit

Participant Preparation

Knowledge Preparation:
- Review the pathophysiology and clinical manifestations of COPD

Skill Preparation:
- Assessment, with a focus on respiratory and cardiovascular systems

- Review assessment needed for a patient with COPD
- Review laboratory and diagnostic findings related to the respiratory status of a patient with COPD
- Review safe oxygen delivery methods
- Application of oxygen delivery systems
- Medication administration, including inhaled route

Evidence-Based Practice Recommendations

1. All individuals identified as having **dyspnea** related to chronic obstructive pulmonary disease (COPD) will be assessed appropriately, to include: vital signs, respiratory assessment, cardiovascular assessment, and level of consciousness.

2. Nurses will be able to implement appropriate nursing interventions for all levels of dyspnea including acute episodes of respiratory distress. Interventions include safe administration of prescribed medications by various routes, controlled oxygen therapy, breathing strategies to help gas exchange and secretion clearance, activity tolerance plan and nutrition plan.

3. Education for the patient with COPD should include smoking cessation strategies if needed, breathing techniques, meeting nutritional needs, and accurate use of medication and inhaler devices.

4. Health Promotion includes administering pneumococcal vaccine and annual influenza vaccination for individuals without contraindications.

Are You Ready?

1. What questions would you ask a patient to assess for breathing difficulty?

2. What would you expect a patient to look like who is short of breath?

3. How would you administer medications that help open narrowed airways?

4. What are your priority nursing actions for a patient with **hypoxia**?

Continue on to meet the patient!

Patient Information

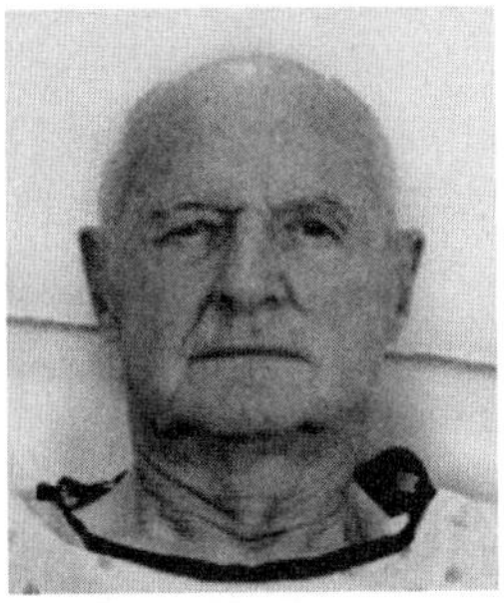

Name	Medical Record Number	Birth Date	Allergies
Henry Winston	101-33-986	12/14/1933	Sulfonamides
Height	**Weight**	**Gender**	**Attending Physician**
65 inches	185 lbs	Male	Dr. Han Lee

Past Medical History

Previously diagnosed with emphysema. History of **MI**, **HTN**, Left-sided **heart failure**, fractured ankle.

Initial Vital Signs

T 98.4°F, P 88, R 20, B/P 126/84, SpO_2 93% **RA** on admit, Pain 4/10 with cough

? **Clinical Competency**

1. What is your interpretation of the patient's vital signs?

Physician Orders

Oxygen to maximum 4 L/min to keep pulse oximetry ≥ 90%
Prednisolone 80 mg po q day
Aspirin 81 mg po daily
Atrovent (ipratropium bromide) 2 puffs t.i.d.
Albuterol MDI 2 puffs q 6 hr prn
Lasix (furosemide) 40 mg po daily
Lopressor (metoprolol) 50 mg po bid
Lanoxin (digoxin) 0.125 mg po daily
CXR, CBC, Chem 7, Chem 15, ABGs, UA
Low sodium (4 gram) diet
Up with assistance
VS q 4 hours and prn
Saline lock
I/O

? **Clinical Competency**

2. Why is each medication prescribed for this patient?
3. Is each medication safe to administer to this patient?
4. What are concerns the nurse has with administering oxygen at a high flow rate to this patient?

Nurse Report

Henry Winston is a married male whose DOB is 12/14/1933, admitted after midnight with acute exacerbation of COPD. Assessment reveals an anxious man who is becoming more dyspneic with exertion. The **UAP** just got a pulse oximetry of 88% on RA. He does not use oxygen at home. Heart rate is regular. Respirations are labored, with right lower lobe crackles and wheezing bilaterally. He is up with assist but he is voiding per urinal as he does not tolerate getting up to the bathroom. Saline lock is in place and patent.

S Increased SOB
B 70 pack-year history of smoking. Complaint of increased dyspnea at home for past 24 hours. Exhibiting increased SOB and his **SpO_2** is now 88% on RA. **ABG**s and labs were drawn, results just arrived
A Worsening respiratory distress and hypoxia

R Assess respiratory status, evaluate ABG results, initiate oxygen therapy and position patient as needed

S Falls Risk
B Ambulates independently with fairly steady gait
A Increasing SOB, weakness
R Implement fall precautions and ambulation with assist

Additional Information

Paternal history of **CAD**.
Hx of smoking 2 packs per day but quit recently
Drinks 2 beers/week
Married, 1 child

? **Clinical Competency**

5. ***What is the primary problem for this patient?***
6. ***What are your priority assessments for this patient?***
7. ***What would you do first for this patient?***

References

Agency for Healthcare Research and Quality (2005). Guideline Summary COPD. U.S. Department of Health & Human Services: Rockville, MD.

Deglin, J.H., Vallerand, A.H., & Sanoski, C.A. (2010). *Davis's Drug Guide for Nurses* (12th ed). F.A. Davis Company: Philadelphia, PA.

Venes, D. (Ed.). (2009). *Taber's Cyclopedic Medical Dictionary* (21st ed). Philadelphia, PA: F.A. Davis Company.

Wilkinson, J.M. & Leuven K.V. (2007). *Fundamentals of Nursing: Theory, Concepts, & Applications.* Philadelphia, PA: F.A. Davis Co.

Williams, L.S. & Hopper, P.D. (2007). *Understanding Medical-Surgical Nursing* (3rd ed). Philadelphia, PA: F.A. Davis Co.

Hip Fracture
Student Information

Introduction

This simulation presents a Caucasian male whose DOB is 02/23/1944, with a left **hip fracture**. Surgical repair was needed to reduce and stabilize the fracture. The surgeon performed an **Open Reduction and Internal Fixation** (ORIF). The participants will manage the postoperative patient and recognize abnormal assessment findings.

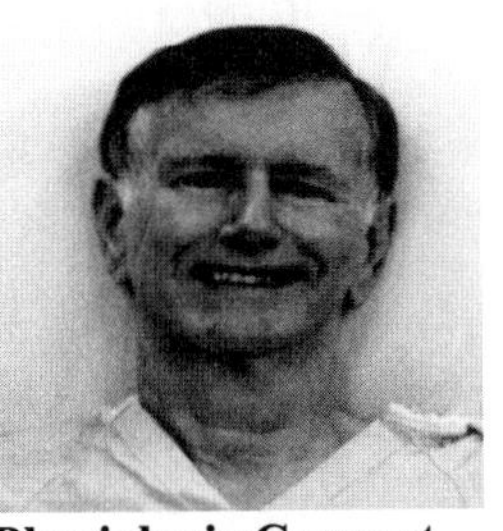

Physiologic Concept

Musculoskeletal

Medical Diagnosis

A hip fracture occurs when there is a break in the continuity of the bone of the femur. The fracture can occur in the head, neck, intertrochanteric region or subtrochanteric region of the femur. There are 2 classifications for hip fractures, intracapsular and extracapsular. Intracapsular fractures occur in the neck of the femur. This type of fracture has an increased risk of sustaining damage to the vascular system. This can result in a decreased blood supply to the head of the femur. Extracapsular fractures occur in the trochanteric regions. This type of fracture usually has a good blood supply and heals quickly.

Hip fractures are common in older adults and often occur from falling. Older adults have a decrease in bone mass, decreased mobility, and other medical problems such as osteoporosis and cardiovascular disease. As a person ages, the risk for falling increases. Poor vision, neurological disorders, orthostatic hypotension, musculoskeletal dysfunction, and environmental hazards often contribute to falls that result in a hip fracture. Many older people have a higher risk of experiencing complications after a hip fracture because of stress related to the trauma and immobility. For older patients many of these complications can result in death. Common clinical manifestations seen when a person has a hip fracture are shortening of the affected extremity, pain, tenderness, external rotation, adduction, and muscle spasms.

Traction can be used to stabilize the fracture in some patients. Surgical treatment is often performed to obtain fixation of the fractured bone and to promote mobilization. Providing nursing care for a postoperative hip fracture patient can be challenging. Nursing care should be directed toward promoting comfort, maintaining circulation in the affected leg, improving mobility, and preventing secondary medical problems from occurring.

Learning Objectives

- ✓ Describe secondary diagnosis which may contribute to hip replacement
- ✓ Identify interview questions for patients with hip fracture postoperatively
- ✓ Conduct a focused assessment on the patient with hip fracture postoperatively
- ✓ Identify specific patient needs and prioritize outcome criteria
- ✓ Intervene to assist patient in achieving identified outcomes
- ✓ Evaluate patient status following care
- ✓ Document all aspects of patient care

Simulation Setting

Adult Patient Orthopedic Unit

Participant Preparation

Knowledge Preparation:

- Review pathophysiology and clinical manifestations of Hip Fracture
- Review assessment needed for the postoperative Hip Fracture patient
- Review oxygen delivery methods for a postoperative Hip Fracture patient
- Review nursing care for the postoperative hip fracture patient
- Review laboratory and diagnostic findings related to for the postoperative Hip Fracture patient
- Review pain management for the postoperative Hip Fracture patient

Skill Preparation:

- Assessment of all body systems
- Medication administration
- Application of oxygen delivery systems
- Measurement of oxygen saturation levels
- Pain assessment and management
- Surgical wound: assessment and dressing change

Evidence-Based Practice Recommendations

1. All individuals identified as a posteroperative hip fracture patient will be assessed appropriately. An assessment of all body sytems must be conducted. Assessment should include VS, breath sounds, pulse oximetry, intake/output, skin turgor, fatigue, dyspnea, bowel sounds, level of consciousness peripheral edema, pedal pulses, restlessness, and pain. The affected leg should be assessed for temperature, warmth, and circulation. The wound should be assessed for size, color, and signs of infection.

2. Nurses will be able to implement interventions for a postoperative hip fracture patient. Interventions should include monitoring VS, monitoring managing pain, giving medications as ordered, encouraging distraction, promoting exercise, applying anti-embolism stockings or a pneumatic compression device, encouraging to participate in physical therapy, repositioning, applying hip abduction pillow when in bed, obtaining oxygen saturation, adminstering oxygen therapy as ordered, as well as monitoring and managing potential complications.

3. Patient education will be provided to assist the patient in understanding the disease process, exercise program to improve mobility and bone density, wound management, and signs of infection. Education should also be provided to improve the knowledge of all medications.

4. Health promotion will be encouraged by providing information regarding preventing falls and removing hazards in the home. Promoting independence is very important. Follow-up appointments should be encouraged. The patient should also understand dietary requirements, be encouraged to participate in an exercise program, identify signs of infection, and know the importance of monitoring blood pressure.

Are You Ready?

1. What would you expect a postoperative hip fracture patient to look like?
2. What is involved for a wound assessment?
3. What questions would you ask the patient regarding his or her home environment?
4. What circulatory changes is the patient at risk for developing in the affected leg?
5. What are your priority nursing interventions for a new postoperative patient?

Continue on to meet the patient!

Simulation: 2 **Hip Fracture**

Patient Information

Name	Medical Record Number	Birth Date	Allergies
Larry Bailey	224-86-983	02/23/1944	Sulfa drugs Allergic to strawberries

Height	Weight	Gender	Attending Physician
65 in	135 lbs	Male	Dr. Han Lee

Past Medical History

Hypertension
Hyperlipidemia

Initial Vital Signs

Vital signs: T 100.0°F, P 90, R 20, BP120/95, SpO2 95% RA, Pain 6/10

? **Clinical Competency**

1. ***What is your interpretation of the vital signs?***
2. ***What circulatory responses should the nurse assess for when a patient has a hip fracture?***

Physician Orders

Oxygen O_2 **2L**/min per **NC**; titrate to keep $\mathbf{O_2}$ sat > 94% (O_2 max. 5L/min)
Morphine Sulfate 2 **mg IV q** 2 hours prn
Zocor (simvastatin) 40 mg po daily
Micardis (telmisartan) 12.5 mg po daily
Tylenol (acetaminophen) 650 mg po q 4 hours prn
Lovenox (enoxaparin) 30 mg **subcut qd**
Saline lock
Saline flush q shift
Ice chips, progress to clear liquids
Hip abductor pillow
Incentive spirometry

? **Clinical Competency**

3. ***Why is each medication prescribed for this patient?***
4. ***Is each medication safe to administer to this patient?***

Nurse Report

Larry Bailey is a male whose DOB is 02/23/1944, who fell off of a step stool and was unable to get up. His daughter found him on the floor and called an ambulance. In the emergency room he was diagnosed with a left hip fracture. An ORIF was performed in surgery. He is alert and oriented X3. Breathing is regular and non-labored. His lungs are clear bilaterally but diminished in the bases. Mr. Bailey has not had a bowel movement since he had surgery. He is uncomfortable and states the pain level in his left hip is 6/10.

S Left hip fracture, immediately post-op
B History of hyperlipidemia and hypertension
A Left hip fracture
R Physical therapy to assist patient to chair. Hip abductor pillow as needed. Monitor incision site.

Additional Information

Cigarettes: None. Never smoked.
Alcohol: Glass of wine with dinner on outings.
Marital Status: Married with one child
Paternal hx of lung cancer
Maternal hx of Cerebral Vascular Accident

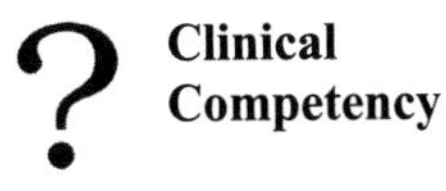

5. What is your primary problem for this patient?

References

Agency for Healthcare Research and Quality (2009). Management of hip fracture in older people: A national clinical guideline. U.S. Department of Health & Human Services: Rockville, MD.

Deglin, J.H., Vallerand, A.H., & Sanoski, C.A. (2010). *Davis's Drug Guide for Nurses* (12th ed). F.A. Davis Company: Philadelphia, PA.

Venes, D. (Ed.). (2009). *Taber's Cyclopedic Medical Dictionary* (21st ed.). Philadelphia, PA: F.A. Davis Company.

Wilkinson, J.M. & Leuven K.V. (2007). *Fundamentals of Nursing: Theory, Concepts, & Applications.* Philadelphia, PA: F.A. Davis Co.

Williams, L.S. & Hopper, P.D. (2007). *Understanding Medical-Surgical Nursing* (3rd ed). Philadelphia, PA: F.A. Davis Co.

Dementia
Student Information

Introduction

This simulation presents a female patient whose DOB is 05/25/1932, admitted with acute confusion related to dementia of the **Alzheimer's** type. The client presents with a chief complaint of confusion reported by the husband. The participants will manage the patient's signs and symptoms, and plan for discharge care, based on assessment findings.

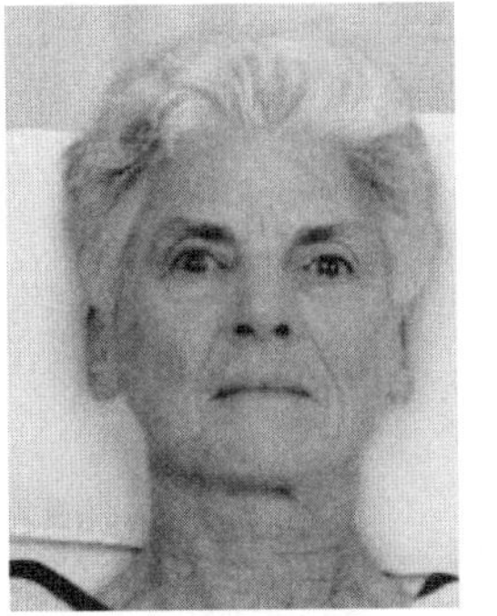

Physiologic Concept

Cognitive Impairment

Medical Diagnosis

Dementia is a loss of brain function that occurs with certain diseases such as Alzheimer's disease (AD), HIV-associated dementia, or Huntington's disease. Dementia affects memory, thinking, language, judgment, and behavior. All forms of dementia result from the death of nerve cells and/or the loss of communication among these cells. Abnormal protein structures or genetic abnormalities may play a role in developing dementia.

Risk factors for developing dementia include advancing age, family history, smoking and alcohol use (increases the development of atherosclerosis), high cholesterol, diabetes (increases atherosclerosis and stroke risk), head injury and Down syndrome.

Symptoms of dementia include memory loss, inability to remember the correct word desired, confusion even in familiar surroundings, frustration from not remembering, change in sleep patterns, mood swings, difficulty doing basic tasks such as dressing, and inability to balance a checkbook. As dementia progresses, the patient can no longer understand language, recognize family members, perform **ADL**s, have difficulty swallowing, and become incontinent. Safety concerns are a high priority for the patient with dementia, both in the hospital and in the home setting.

Medications used in treating Alzheimer's disease slow the progression of the disease but do not reverse existing brain damage. Cognitive symptoms of AD are treated with cholinesterase inhibitors to improve quality of life and cognitive functions including memory, thought and reasoning. Memantine may also be used to improve learning and memory. Anticonvulsants, sedatives and antidepressants may also be prescribed to treat problems associated with dementia.

Learning Objectives

- ✓ Identify signs and symptoms of dementia
- ✓ Identify interview questions for the dementia patient and caregivers
- ✓ Conduct a focused assessment on the patient with dementia:
  - a) Evaluate safety factors
  - b) Evaluate diagnostic and laboratory findings
  - c) Evaluate self-care factors
  - d) Perform basic mental status assessment and organize results and observations
- ✓ Identify specific patient needs and prioritize outcome criteria
- ✓ Intervene to assist patient in achieving identified outcomes
- ✓ Evaluate patient status following care
- ✓ Document all aspects of patient care

Simulation Setting

Adult Patient Medical Unit

Participant Preparation

Knowledge Preparation:

- Review the pathophysiology and clinical manifestations of dementia
- Review possible treatments for a patient with dementia
- Review safety issues that should be initiated in the hospital related to a patient who is confused
- Review needs for a caregiver with a confused family member

Skill Preparation:

- Assessment, with a focus on neurologic system, including a mental status exam
- Medication administration
- Communication skills with a confused patient
- Develop discharge plan

Evidence-Based Practice Recommendations

1. A patient with dementia requires ongoing evaluation of physical and mental status. Monitoring of routine diagnostic tests is also part of assessment. Safety issues are an ongoing concern.

2. Nursing interventions strive to meet ADL and safety issues of the patient. Behavior modification, such as scheduled toileting, prompted voiding to reduce urinary incontinence. Music during meals and bathing has been shown to be effective. Walking or other light activity helps reduce behavior problems. Caregiver training is a critical part of case management.

3. Education focuses on family/caregiver training to meet the needs of the patient. Safe administration of medications, meeting nutritional needs, sleep needs and safety needs are priority needs for the patient. Referral to the Alzheimer's Association is recommended. The home environment needs adaptations to provide for the safety of a patient with dementia. For example, sharp knives, scissors, etc. need to be placed in a safe place. Safety bars can be installed in the bedroom and bathroom. Water heater temperatures should be set at 120° or less. The patient should wear some form of identification at all times, and door alarms can be installed. Caregiver strain should also be monitored.

   Health promotion includes regular health screening and scheduled immunizations.

Are You Ready?

1. What behaviors would you expect the patient with dementia to exhibit?

2. How can you provide a safe environment for the patient with dementia?

3. How can you help a patient with confusion feel safe while in the hospital?

4. How do you administer a mental status exam? How are the results used?

5. What are the legal/ethical issues surrounding the use of physical restraints in a patient with dementia?

6. How can you support the caregiver of a family member with dementia?

Continue on to meet the patient!

Simulation: 3

Dementia

Patient Information

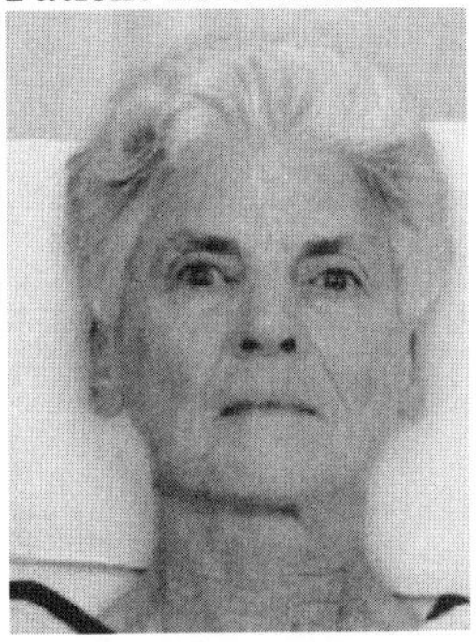

Name	Medical Record Number	Birth Date	Allergies
Hazel Boatman	374-82-234	05/25/1942	NKDA, no known food allergies, allergy to cats

Height	Weight	Gender	Attending Physician
67 inches	135 lbs	Female	Dr. Han Lee

Past Medical History

Hx of **hypothyroidism**.

Initial Vital Signs

T 99°F, P 68, R 16, B/P 114/68, SpO_2 95% on **RA**, pain 0/10

? **Clinical Competency**

1. ***What is your interpretation of the patient's vital signs?***

Physician Orders

Donepezil (Aricept) 10 mg po **HS**
Memantine (Namenda) 10 mg po q am
Multi-vitamin 1 po q am
Docusate (Colace) 100 mg po bid
Synthroid (Levothyroxine sodium) 0.1 mg po q day
Fall precautions
Up with assist only
Diet as tolerated, encourage fluids
CT of head in am
CBC, Chem 7, Chem 15, **UA**
Vitals q 4 hrs
Social services referral for home assist, placement needs
Calorie count, **I/O**

? **Clinical Competency**

2. ***Why is each medication prescribed for this patient?***
3. ***Is each medication safe to administer to this patient?***
4. ***What medication administration problems may arise in a patient who is confused?***

Nurse Report

Hazel Boatman is a female whose DOB is 05/25/1932, admitted last night at 2300 from home for altered mental status. Husband reports that over the past two days, she has become increasingly confused, agitated and had attempted to leave the home unclothed. She also set the kitchen stove on fire when she placed a towel in the oven. Vital signs are stable. Heart is regular, lung sounds clear. She is oriented to person only. Bowel sounds are hypoactive. Appetite is poor. She had 100 mL intake and 200 mL voided urine over the last shift.

S Altered mental status
B Worsening over last 2 days per primary caregiver (husband)
A Altered mental status, likely dementia
R Assess mental status through patient interview. Review lab results, document patient care

S Falls risk
B Ambulates independently but altered mental status creates wander and fall risk
A Altered mental status, likely dementia
R Implement falls precautions

Additional Information

Family hx of maternal major depressive disorder. Has never smoked, drinks 1–2 glasses of wine/week

? **Clinical Competency**

5. ***What is the primary problem for this patient?***
6. ***What are your priority assessments for this patient?***
7. ***What would you do first for this patient?***
8. ***How can you meet the safety needs for this patient?***

References

Agency for Healthcare Research and Quality (2009). Guideline summary management of patients with dementia. U.S. Department of Health & Human Services: Rockville, MD.

Deglin, J.H., Vallerand, A.H., & Sanoski, C.A. (2010). *Davis's Drug Guide for Nurses* (12th ed.). Philadelphia, PA: F.A. Davis Company

Detection, diagnosis and management of dementia, (n.d.). American Academy of Neurology, St. Paul, MN. Retrieved August 1, 2010 from http://www.aan.com/professionals/practice/-pdfs/dementia_guideline.pdf

Venes, D. (Ed.). (2009). *Taber's Cyclopedic Medical Dictionary*. Philadelphia, PA: F.A. Davis Company.

Wilkinson, J.M. & Leuven K.V. (2007). *Fundamentals of Nursing: Theory, Concepts, & Applications.* Philadelphia, PA: F.A. Davis Co.

Williams, L.S. & Hopper, P.D. (2007). *Understanding Medical-Surgical Nursing* (3rd ed). Philadelphia, PA: F.A. Davis Co.

Heart Failure
Student Information

Introduction

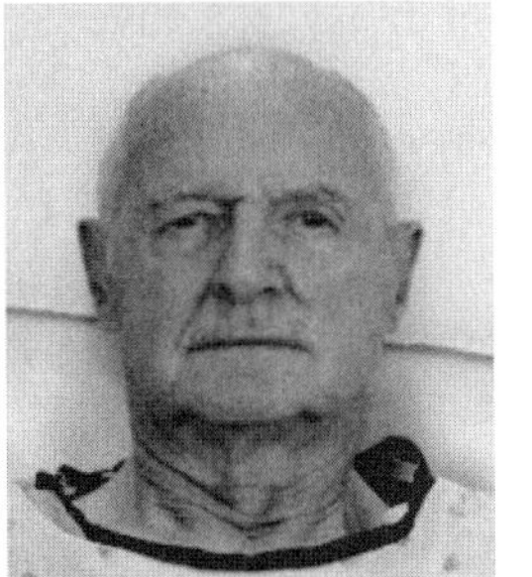

This simulation presents a male patient whose DOB is 12/14/1933, admitted with **heart failure**, also called congestive heart failure (**CHF**). The client presents with a chief complaint of fatigue.
The participants will manage the patient's signs and symptoms based on assessment findings

Physiologic Concept

Oxygenation, Perfusion

Medical Diagnosis

Heart failure, also called congestive heart failure (CHF), is a condition in which the heart can no longer pump enough oxygen-rich blood to the rest of the body. The condition may affect the right and/or left side of the heart.

Major risk factors for heart failure include heart attack, **HTN**, **CAD**, and heart valve disease. Other causes include cardiac infections, **diabetes mellitus**, smoking, alcohol abuse, increased oxygen needs, and congenital defects.

Weakened heart muscles in heart failure result in decreased ejection of blood to the body, which affects many organs of the body. Decreased perfusion to the kidneys may result in a decreased ability to excrete salt (sodium) and water, leading to fluid retention. Fluids accumulate in the lungs, liver, and intestines, impairing their function. Fluid also accumulates in the extremities, resulting in **edema** (swelling) of the arms, hands, ankles and feet.

Common symptoms of heart failure include: shortness of breath with activity or at rest, cough, swelling of feet and ankles, swelling of the abdomen, weight gain from fluid retention, irregular or rapid pulse, sensation of feeling the heart beat (palpitations), difficulty sleeping, fatigue, weakness, faintness, loss of appetite, indigestion, and decreased urine production.

Medications are typically needed in the treatment of heart failure to improve heart function and eliminate excess fluid. Necessary lifestyle changes include smoking cessation, limiting salt intake, weight loss as needed, and a monitored exercise program.

Learning Objectives

- ✓ Differentiate between the clinical manifestations of right and left sided heart failure
- ✓ Recognize signs of decreased cardiac output to include fatigue, **SOB**, additional sounds that are heard over normal breath sounds, peripheral edema and impaired urinary elimination
- ✓ Identify interview questions for the patient with CHF
- ✓ Conduct a focused assessment on the patient with CHF
- ✓ Check medications administration according to MAR
- ✓ Evaluate the effectiveness of treatment for a patient with excess fluid volume
- ✓ Document patient response to care

Simulation Setting

Adult Patient Medical Unit

Participant Preparation

Knowledge Preparation:

- Review the pathophysiology and clinical manifestations of right and left-sided heart failure
- Review assessment needed for a patient with cardiac and respiratory illness
- Review laboratory and diagnostic findings related to the patient with heart failure
- Review common medications prescribed for heart failure
- Review safe oxygen delivery methods

Skill Preparation:

- Assessment, with a focus on respiratory and cardiovascular systems
- Application of oxygen delivery systems
- Medication administration

Evidence-Based Practice Recommendations

1. Assessment for patients with heart failure should focus on the cardiovascular and respiratory systems. Patient history should include assessment of smoking history, alcohol use, and ability to perform routine tasks.

2. Nursing interventions appropriate for the patient with heart failure include I/O, oxygen therapy, administration of prescribed medications, monitoring of diagnostic tests, activity management, daily weight, and vital signs with pulse oximetry

3. Education includes teaching for any diet and fluid restrictions, activity limitations, prescribed medications, and symptoms to report weight gain, shortness of breath, cough, fatigue, edema, chest pain, and dizziness. It is very important the patient keep follow-up appointments with a health care provider.

4. Health promotion activities need to address smoking cessation counseling if indicated, annual influenza vaccine and pneumococcal vaccine when due unless contraindicated.

Are You Ready?

1. What questions would you ask to assess the respiratory and cardiac status of your patient?

2. How would you perform a focused cardiovascular assessment?

3. What are interventions for **hypoxia**? For patients with systemic signs of edema?

4. What do you expect to see in a patient with heart failure?

Continue on to meet the patient!

Simulation: 4

Heart Failure

Patient Information

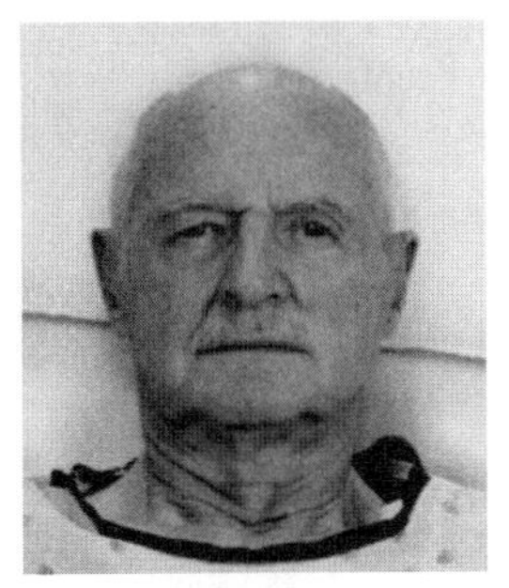

Name	Medical Record Number	Birth Date	Allergies
Henry Winston	100-34-760	12/14/1933	PCN

Height	Weight	Gender	Attending Physician
65 inches	160 lbs	Male	Dr. Han Lee

Past Medical History

Previously diagnosed with **MI**, **HTN**, Left-sided **heart failure**

Initial Vital Signs

T 97.8°F, P 92, R 20, B/P 154/86, **SpO_2** 94% on room air, Pain 0/10

? **Clinical Competency**

1. What is your interpretation of the patient's vital signs?

Physician Orders

Oxygen to maximum 4 L/min to keep pulse oximetry ≥ 90%
Vital signs q 4 hours with pulse oximetry
Lab: CBC, UA, chem 7, chem 15, CXR
Lasix (furosemide) 40 mg po daily
Lanoxin (digoxin) 0.125 mg po daily
Vasotec (enalapril) 10 mg po daily
Lopressor (metoprolol) 50 mg po twice a day
Potassium chloride 20 mEq po twice a day
Saline lock
No added salt diet
Restrict fluids to 2000 mL/24 hours
Bed rest
Daily weight
EKG from ED on chart
I/O

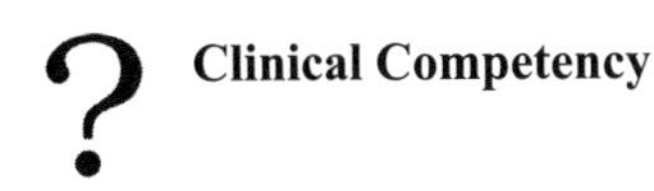

Clinical Competency

2. Why is each medication prescribed for this patient?
3. Is each medication safe to administer to this patient?
4. How are signs and symptoms for right-sided heart failure different from left-sided heart failure?

Nurse Report

Henry Winston is a widowed male whose DOB is 12/14/1933, admitted 2 days ago with exacerbation of heart failure. He has a **hx** of MI, HTN and heart failure. His current medications are for these conditions. He has not been on oxygen since last night. He is alert and oriented, on a no added salt diet and 2000 mL fluid restriction. Patient is currently complaining of increasing SOB and cough. The last pulse ox was 94% on room air 2 hours ago. Lungs are diminished with wheeze audible bilaterally. Heart rate is slightly irregular. He has DOE and is on bed rest. 2+ peripheral edema is present. Weight this morning is 169 lbs, up 9 pounds from baseline. Abdomen is distended with hypoactive bowel sounds. Saline lock is in place. We have had trouble with the low sodium diet and fluid restriction, as he has been having a family member bring in carbonated beverages from home, but he has not been eating his meals here because he is not hungry. Labs just came back.

S CHF exacerbation
B Hx of heart failure and noncompliance with diet. Hx of HTN, MI. On multiple medications.

A SOB r/t fluid retention and pulmonary edema. Peripheral edema present. **Anorexia.**
R Assess for increased respiratory distress, review **I/O**. Treat hypoxia and document care

Additional Information

Paternal hx of coronary vascular disease.
Hx of smoking 1 packs per day but quit long ago
Drinks 2 beers/week
Widower, 2 children

? **Clinical Competency**

5. ***What is the primary problem for this patient?***
6. ***What are your priority assessments for this patient?***
7. ***What would you do first for this patient?***

References

Jessup, M. (2009). 2009 Focused update: ACCF/AHA Guidelines for the diagnosis and management of heart failure in adults. Circulation, 119, 1977–2016.
Deglin, J.H., Vallerand, A.H., & Sanoski, C.A. (2010). *Davis's Drug Guide for Nurses* (12th ed). F.A. Davis Company: Philadelphia, PA.
Venes, D. (Ed.). (2009). *Taber's Cyclopedic Medical Dictionary* (21st ed.). Philadelphia, PA: F.A. Davis Company.
Wilkinson, J.A., et al. (2010). *Fundamentals of Nursing*. Philadelphia, PA: F.A. Davis Co.
Williams, L.S. & Hopper, P.D. (2007). *Understanding Medical-Surgical Nursing* (3rd ed). Philadelphia, PA: F.A. Davis Co.

Small Bowel Obstruction
Student Information

Introduction

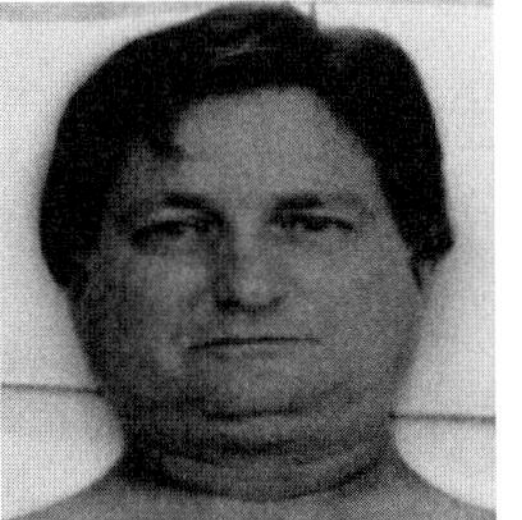

This simulation presents a Caucasian male whose DOB is 09/14/1967, with a **Small Bowel Obstruction (SBO)**. The patient presents with decreased bowel sounds, nausea, vomiting, and severe upper abdominal pain. The participants will manage the signs and symptoms based on assessment findings.

Physiologic Concept

Elimination

Medical Diagnosis

A Small Bowel Obstruction (SBO) is an obstruction that occurs in the small intestine. An **Intestinal obstruction** occurs when intestinal contents are partially or completely blocked and the normal flow is interrupted. Gas, fluid, and intestinal contents, will have difficulty moving through the intestinal track. This results in retention of fluids and abdominal distention. Absorption will be decreased and the production for more gastric contents will be stimulated. This will continue to decrease intestinal motility. Abdominal distention and pressure in the abdomen will continue to increase. This can result in congestion, edema, necrosis, and perforation of the intestinal wall. A large amount of fluid can remain in the intestinal track resulting in dehydration, electrolyte imbalances, **hypovolemia**, and shock. Intestinal obstructions are caused by hernias, benign or cancerous tumors, inflammatory bowel diseases, diverticular disease, volvulus, and paralytic ileus.

Patients often present with abdominal distention, abdominal pain, vomiting, rectal bleeding, and a change in bowel elimination pattern. The severity of an intestinal obstruction can vary. Factors that can influence the severity include the area of the affected bowel, the extent to which the lumen is occluded, and the extent of disturbance to the bowel wall caused by decreased vascular supply.

Treatment is given to relieve the obstruction and restore normal bowel function. Initially the patient is placed on **NPO** status and decompression of the bowel is needed. The insertion of a **nasogastric (NG)** tube is often used to decompress the bowel. Surgery is often needed if the patient's condition does not improve in 24–48 hours.

Learning Objectives

- ✓ Perform an abdominal assessment including: Auscultation of bowel sounds and palpation of abdomen for masses
- ✓ Obtain a thorough history of bowel elimination
- ✓ Assess abdominal pain
- ✓ Maintain **NPO** status and monitor IV therapy: Intake and output and IV flow rate
- ✓ Perform NG insertion: Instruct patient about need for NG and procedure prior to insertion
- ✓ Provide oral hygiene
- ✓ Document all aspects of patient care

Simulation Setting

Adult Patient Medical Unit

Participant Preparation

Knowledge Preparation:

- Review the pathophysiology and clinical manifestations of SBO
- Review assessment needed for the patient with a SBO
- Review the procedure for inserting and maintaining the function of a NG tube
- Review the procedure for administering and maintaining IV fluids
- Review laboratory and diagnostic findings for a SBO

Skill Preparation:

- Assessment with a focus on the gastrointestinal system
- Medication administration
- Assess IV site and administer IV fluids ordered
- Prepare to insert a NG tube

Evidence-Based Practice Recommendations

1. All individuals identified as having a SBO will be assessed appropriately. The nurse should obtain vital signs, conduct a gastrointestinal assessment, and review diagnostic laboratory results.
2. Nurses will be able to implement appropriate interventions for SBO. Nursing interventions should include monitoring all laboratory and diagnostic results, insertion and maintance of a NG tube, monitoring fluid and electrolyte imbalances, maintaing nutrition, monitoring elimination pattern, montoring abdominal girth, providing comfort measures, and if needed prepare the patient for surgery.
3. Education for the patient with a SBO should include information on the disease process, monitoring bowel elimination pattern, meeting nutrition needs, making a list of signs and symptoms if they have elimination problems in the future, and seeing the doctor immediately if they think this problem has developed again.
4. Health promotion includes the importance of maintaining follow-up appointments, increasing fiber intake, increasing fluid intake, and exercising.

Are You Ready?

1. What would you expect a patient to look like who is experiecing a SBO?
2. What signs and symptoms would the nurse assess for in a patient with a SBO?
3. What questions would you ask the patient regarding their bowel elimination pattern?
4. What are your priority nursing interventions for a patient with a SBO?

Continue on to meet the patient!

Patient Information

Name	Medical Record Number	Birth Date	Allergies
Colin Bloch	528-65-290	09/14/1967	NKDA

Height	Weight	Gender	Attending Physician
6 ft	172 lbs	Male	Dr. Han Lee

Past Medical History

Crohn's disease
Subtotal colectomy
Colitis exacerbation
Acute abdominal pain
Colitis/**hematochezia**

Initial Vital Signs

T 97.8F, P 88, R 20, BP125/84, SpO2 94% RA, Pain 9/10

? **Clinical Competency**

1. ***What is your interpretation of the vital signs?***
2. ***What factors put Mr. Bloch at risk for developing a bowel obstruction?***

Physician Orders

Mesalamine (Apriso) 800 **mg po bid**
Omeprazole (Prilosec) 20 mg po **qd**
Hyoscyamine (Anaspaz) 0.25 mg **IV** q**6h** prn intestinal cramping
Morphine Sulfate 1.5 mg IV q 3–4 hrs prn pain
D_5 0.45 % NaCl @100**mL**/hr
NPO
NG tube to low intermittent suction
Insert foley catheter on call to surgery
Bedrest
VS q4h
Monitor intake/output
Abdominal x-ray

? **Clinical Competency**

3. ***Why is each medication prescribed for this patient?***
4. ***Is each medication safe to administer to this patient?***

Nurse Report

Colin Bloch is a male whose DOB is 09/14/1967, admitted this morning with a SBO. He has a history of Crohn's disease. Assessment reveals he has not had a bowel movement in a couple of days. He has a distended abdomen, abdominal pain, nausea, and vomiting. Mr. Bloch states he has been experiencing nausea and vomiting for the last 14 hours.

S Decreased/absent bowel sounds auscultated throughout distended abdomen
B Nausea and vomiting for 14 hrs prior to admission, insert NG tube and connect to low intermittent suction ordered, IV D_5 0.45% NaCl at 100mL/hr
A Continuing decreased/absent bowel sounds with SBO
R Insert NG tube to low intermittent suction and elevate **HOB** to 45 degrees, monitor **I/O**

S Abdominal pain
B SBO, has not received morphine yet this morning
A Ongoing abdominal pain
R Assess and treat pain as ordered, position for comfort PRN, document care

S Nausea and vomiting
B SBO, History of Crohn's disease
A Ongoing nausea and vomiting
R Insert NG tube for gastric decompression, assess and treat nausea and vomiting with antiemetic as ordered, document care

Additional Information

Married with no children
Does not smoke cigarettes
Drinks alcohol occasionally

? **Clinical Competency**

5. What is your primary problem for this patient?
6. What are your priority assessments for this patient?

References

Agency for Healthcare Research and Quality (2007). Practice management guidelines for small bowel obstruction. U.S. Department of Health & Human Services: Rockville, MD.

Deglin, J.H., Vallerand, A.H., & Sanoski, C.A. (2010). *Davis's Drug Guide for Nurses* (12th ed). F.A. Davis Company: Philadelphia, PA.

Venes, D. (Ed.). (2009). *Taber's Cyclopedic Medical Dictionary* (21st ed.). Philadelphia, PA: F.A. Davis Company.

Wilkinson, J.M. & Leuven K.V. (2007). *Fundamentals of Nursing: Theory, Concepts, & Applications.* Philadelphia, PA: F.A. Davis Co.

Williams, L.S. & Hopper, P.D. (2007). *Understanding Medical-Surgical Nursing* (3rd ed). Philadelphia, PA: F.A. Davis Co.

Diabetes Mellitus
Student Information

Introduction

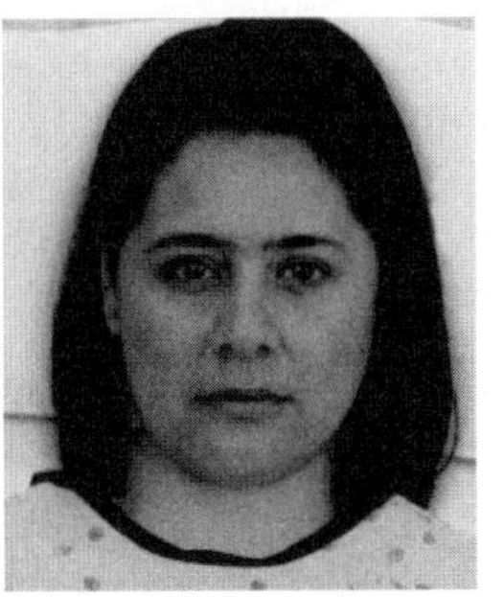

This simulation presents a Hispanic female patient whose DOB is 05/26/1972, admitted with **Diabetic Ketoacidosis (DKA).** On admission, the patient presents with a blood glucose level of 358, fruity breath (acetone breath), and abdominal pain. The participants will manage the signs and symptoms based on assessment findings.

Physiologic Concept

Endocrine, Metabolic, Fluid & Electrolyte

Medical Diagnosis

Diabetes Mellitus (DM) is a chronic autoimmune disorder characterized by **hyperglycemia**. Diabetes Mellitus is a disorder of glucose metabolism and it occurs when there is a defect in insulin secretion, impaired **insulin** utilization or both. People who have diabetes have difficulty converting food to energy.

Type 1 Diabetes Mellitus, **Type 2 Diabetes Mellitus**, and G**estational Diabetes** are major classifications of DM. Type 1 Diabetes Mellitus was formerly known as **juvenile diabetes**, commonly occurs before age 30, has an abrupt onset, and is characterized by a destruction of insulin-secreting beta cells of the pancreas. In type 1 Diabetes Mellitus, the destruction of insulin-secreting beta cells causes a decrease in insulin production. Type 2 Diabetes Mellitus commonly occurs after age 30. In type 2 Diabetes Mellitus the body does not produce enough insulin or the insulin produced is not utilized. This leads to insulin resistance and impaired insulin secretion. People with type 2 Diabetes Mellitus have a family history of diabetes and are obese. Gestational diabetes often develops late in pregnancy due to a decrease in insulin or hormones during pregnancy. This type of diabetes usually goes away after the baby is born. Common clinical manifestations of all types of diabetes are **polyuria**, **polydipsia**, and **polyphagia**.

Diabetic ketoacidosis is a complication of DM. It often occurs from an absence or significant decrease in insulin. The patients with this diagnosis often experience hyperglycemia, acidosis, electrolyte deficits, and dehydration. Diabetic ketoacidosis is commonly seen in the patient with type 1 Diabetes Mellitus. It can also occur in the patient with type 2 Diabetes Mellitus. It can develop when there is an absence or inadequate amount of insulin. This results in abnormal metabolism of protein, carbohydrate, and fat. Hyperglycemia, acidosis, dehydration, and electrolyte loss are common clinical signs of DKA.

Hyperosmolar Hyperglycemic Nonketotic Syndrome (HHNS) is another complication of DM that can develop. In HHNS hyperglycemia and hyperosmolarity dominate and ketones are absent or minimal in both blood and urine. Patients will often experience severe hyperglycemia, extracellular fluid depletion, and osmotic diuresis. HHNS is often seen in the patient with type 2 Diabetes Mellitus.

Learning Objectives

- ✓ Apply knowledge of disease process and long term effects of diabetes mellitus
- ✓ Recognize signs and symptoms of **hypoglycemia** and hyperglycemia
- ✓ Obtain patient's blood sugar using glucometer
- ✓ Determine insulin needs based on sliding scale insulin orders
- ✓ Identify type of insulin needed for sliding scale cover
- ✓ Administer accurate amount of insulin in an appropriate subcutaneous site
- ✓ Document blood sugar and insulin administration on the Medication Administration Record
- ✓ Document focused assessment findings

Simulation Setting

Adult Patient Medical Unit

Participant Preparation

Knowledge Preparation:

- Review the pathophysiology and clinical manifestations of Diabetes
- Review assessment needed for the patient with Diabetes
- Review clinical manifestations of hypoglycemia, hyperglycemia, and diabetic ketoacidosis
- Review nursing implications for insulin used to treat Diabetes
- Review the procedure for administering and maintaining IV fluids
- Review laboratory and diagnostic findings related to alterations in blood glucoses levels for a patient with Diabetes

Skill Preparation:

- Assessment with a focus on the neurological, musculoskeletal, vascular, mouth, skin, and feet
- Medication administration
- Prepare to respond to hyperglycemic and hypoglycemic reactions
- Demonstrate obtaining a blood glucose reading
- Assess IV site and administer IV fluids as ordered

Evidence-Based Practice Recommendations

1. All individuals identified as having DM will be assessed appropriately. The nurse should obtain vital signs and conduct an aassessment of the cardiovascular, respiratory, neurological, gastrointestinal, musculoskeletal, mouth, skin, and feet.

2. Nurses will be able to implement appropriate interventions for DM. Nursing interventions should include monitoring blood glucose levels, safe administration of prescribed medications, determining saftety needs and employ proper precautions, and develop a nutrition and activity plans. The nurse can also assist with referals for interdiscilinary team members to assist in the management of this medical problem.

5. Diabetes Mellitus is a chronic illness that requires a lot of knowledge to enhance self-management behaviors. Patient education will be provided to increase the knowledge and self-management of this disease.
   - Assist to understand disease process
   - Assist to understand and perform skills needed for long term management
   - Increase knowledge of all medications and diabetic diet
   - Provide information on how to recognize, treatment, and prevent complications of the disease
   - Provide information on how to manage sick days
   - Self care techniques to balance physical activity, stress, diet, blood glucose levels, and medications

6. Health promotion includes good hygiene of the skin, feet, and mouth. The importance of maintaining follow-up appointments, dental examinations, and eye examinations should be encouraged. Patients should understand how to manage food, fluids, and medications when they experience sick days. Information on community support groups should be provided. If insulin injections are required, the patient should be able to demonstrate the procedure to administer an injection. All medications should be taken as prescribed.

Are You Ready?

1. What would you expect a patient to look like who is experiecing DKA?

2. What signs and symptoms would the nurse assess for in a patient with DKA?

3. What questions would you ask the patient regarding blood glucose levels?

4. What are your priority nursing interventions for a patient with DKA?

Continue on to meet the patient!

Patient Information

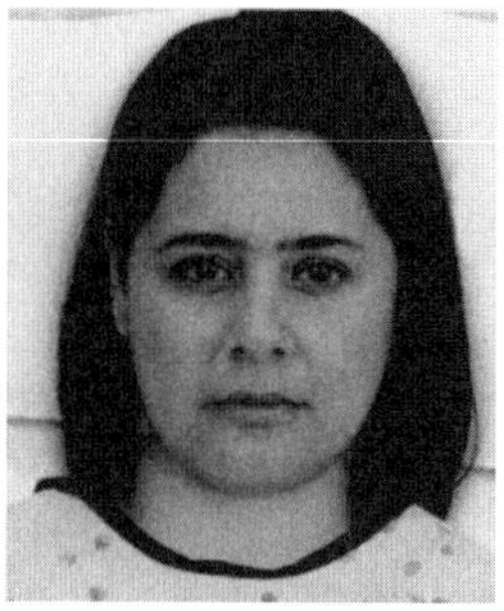

Name	Medical Record Number	Birth Date	Allergies
Maria Hernandez	667-34-987	05/26/1972	Penicillin
Height	**Weight**	**Gender**	**Attending Physician**
5'10"	190 lbs	Female	Dr. Han Lee

Past Medical History

Type 1 Diabetes Mellitus since age 10
Hypertension

Initial Vital Signs

T 97.8°F, P 68, R 18, BP142/88, SpO2 99% RA, Pain 1/10

? **Clinical Competency**

1. What is your interpretation of the vital signs?

Physician Orders

Bedrest
Vital signs **q4h** & prn
Lantus Insulin 20 units **subcut qd** in am
Check the blood sugar (**BS**) before every meal and before bedtime
Regular Insulin per sliding scale

BS=151–200 give 2 Units regular insulin SUBCUT
BS=201–250 give 4 Units regular insulin SUBCUT
BS=251–300 give 6 Units regular insulin SUBCUT
BS=301–350 give 8 Units regular insulin SUBCUT
BS>351 Call the doctor

0.9% **NaCl** 100 mL/hr
Valsartan (diovan) 80 mg po
Potassium chloride 40 **mEq** IV x1
Tylenol (acetaminophen) 325 mg po **q4h** prn
1800 **ADA** Diet
Insert foley catheter

? **Clinical Competency**

2. Why is each medication prescribed for this patient?
3. Is each medication safe to administer to this patient?

Nurse Report

Maria Hernandez is a female whose DOB is 05/26/1972, with a history of Type 1 Diabetes Mellitus who was admitted yesterday with DKA. Her blood sugar has been poorly controlled over the past week. She is awake, alert, and oriented x3. Breathing is regular, deep and nonlabored. She has an IV in the right arm, infusing 0.9% NaCl @ 100 mL. A foley catheter needs to be inserted. Maria states she feels weak and she has some abdominal discomfort.

S Fluctuating blood glucose
B Admitted with blood glucose 358. AM blood glucose 128, 1800 ADA diet ordered
A Unstable blood glucose (diabetes mellitus)
R Monitor blood glucose AC and HS, provide insulin every AM and PRN per sliding scale, monitor 1800ADA diet, assess s/s hyperglycemic and hypoglycemic response

Additional Information

Married with two children
Maternal hyperlipidemia
Does not drink or smoke

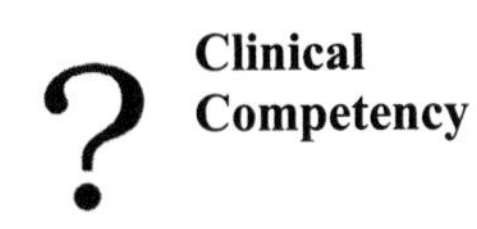

Clinical Competency

4. ***What is your primary problem for this patient?***
5. ***What are your priority assessments for this patient?***
6. ***What are symptoms of hypoglycemia and why is this patient at risk for developing this disorder?***

References

Agency for Healthcare Research and Quality (2009). Guidelines for the practice of diabetes education. U.S. Department of Health & Human Services: Rockville, MD.

Agency for Healthcare Research and Quality (2010). Standards of medical care in diabetes. VI. Prevention and management of diabetes complications. U.S. Department of Health & Human Services: Rockville, MD.

Deglin, J.H., Vallerand, A.H., & Sanoski, C.A. (2010). *Davis's Drug Guide for Nurses* (12th ed). F.A. Davis Company: Philadelphia, PA.

Venes, D. (Ed.). (2009). *Taber's Cyclopedic Medical Dictionary* (21st ed.). Philadelphia, PA: F.A. Davis Company. Co.

Wilkinson, J.M. & Leuven K.V. (2007). *Fundamentals of Nursing: Theory, Concepts, & Applications.* Philadelphia, PA: F.A. Davis Co.

Williams, L.S. & Hopper, P.D. (2007). *Understanding Medical-Surgical Nursing* (3rd ed). Philadelphia, PA: F.A. Davis Co.

Post-Operative Care Post-Mastectomy
Student Information

Introduction

This simulation presents a female Caucasian patient whose DOB is 10/03/1961, admitted for right **mastectomy** as part of her treatment for breast cancer. While the disease process is a specific cancer, there are several principles for post-operative care that are utilized. The participants will manage the patient's post-operative care and assess for psychosocial needs.

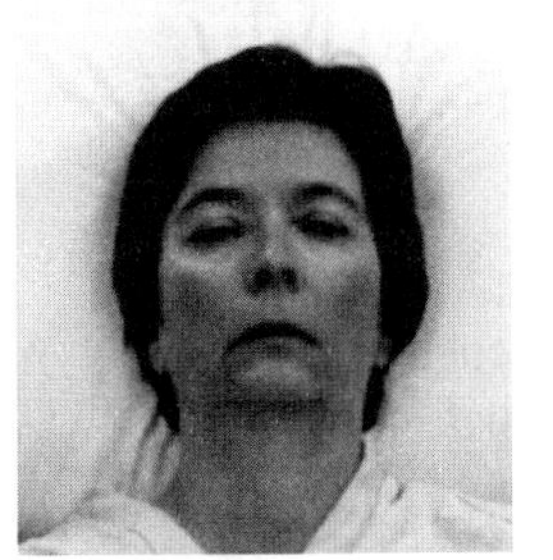

Physiologic Concept

Oxygenation, Infection, Tissue Integrity, Mood /Anxiety

Medical Diagnosis

Breast cancer, the most common form of cancer in women, is a disease in which cells in the breast start to grow abnormally in an uncontrolled manner. Ninety percent of breast cancers occur in women with no family history of the disease; it is so important for all women to get regular mammograms.

Treatment options include chemotherapy, radiation therapy, and surgical options that include lumpectomy and mastectomy. It is important to assist both the patient and their support system in dealing with the stress of the situation/prognosis. It is important to prevent post-operative complications and establish an individualized education and rehabilitation program.

Risk factors for breast cancer include being female, a family history of breast cancer, increasing age, personal history of breast cancer, Caucasian, initiation of menstrual cycle younger than 12 years, menopause older than 55 years of age, and having children later in life. Other risks include a high fat diet, excess alcohol intake, and sedentary lifestyle.

Learning Objectives

- ✓ Assess post-operative incision site
- ✓ Provide drain care
- ✓ Provide pain management
- ✓ Provide emotional support
- ✓ Conduct a focused assessment of a post-surgical patient
- ✓ Identify patient specific needs related to disease process
- ✓ Intervene to assist patient in achieving identified outcomes
- ✓ Evaluate patient status following daily care
- ✓ Document all aspects of patient care

Simulation Setting

Adult Patient Surgical Unit

Participant Preparation

Knowledge Preparation:

- Review the care and assessment for a post-operative patient, including respiratory, circulatory, wound and drain care
- Review assessment needed for a patient with pain and emotional needs

Skill Preparation:

- Assessment, with a focus on musculoskeletal system and skin integrity
- Wound assessment and dressing change
- Care of wound drain
- Administration of pain medication

- Review laboratory and diagnostic findings indicative of post-operative infection

Evidence-Based Practice Recommendations

1. Primary causes for post-operative complications include the surgical wound, the effects of immobilization, effects of anesthesia, and risk factors present prior to surgery. Assessment should focus on identifying any respiratory, cardiac, gastrointestinal and genitourinary, and musculoskeletal systems.

2. Nursing interventions for post-operative care include managing temperature regulation, maintaining neurologic function and fluid and electrolyte balance, promoting elimination, promoting wound healing, and maintaining patient self-concept.

3. Education for a post-operative patient includes measures to prevent post-operative complications, use of pain medications, wound care measures, and discharge instructions. Referrals to appropriate support groups is also important.

4. Health promotion includes ongoing screening appropriate for age and health history and follow-up with health-care providers as needed.

Are You Ready?

1. What is involved for a wound assessment?

2. What care is needed for the patient with post-operative drain tubes? How is drain suction maintained?

3. What mobility issues does a post-mastectomy patient have?

4. How does a nurse perform a pain assessment?

5. What questions does a nurse ask to assess the emotional state of a patient?

6. What does the nurse expect a post-operative patient to look like when the nurse first enters the room?

Continue on to meet the patient!

Patient Information

Name	Medical Record number	Birth Date	Allergies
Victoria Smith	714-09-019	10/03/1961	NKDA
Height	**Weight**	**Gender**	**Attending Physician**
64 inches	170 lbs	Female	Dr. Han Lee

Past Medical History

Diagnosed breast cancer

Initial Vital Signs

T 101.7°F – P 88- R 20- B/P 126/84- **SpO_2** 95% on RA pain 5/10 at incisional site

? **Clinical Competency**

1. ***What is your interpretation of the patient's vital signs?***

Physician Orders

Oxygen to maximum 6 **L**/min to keep pulse oximetry ≥ 92%
Morphine sulfate 2 mg IV q2 h prn.
Tylenol (acetaminophen) 650mg **po** q4 h prn when tolerating diet well
MVI (multivitamin) tab po daily
FeSO4 (ferrous sulfate) 1 tab po daily
Up with assistance **qid**
I/O
Incentive spirometry qid
Vital signs q 4h
Diet as tolerated
Change IV to saline lock

? **Clinical Competency**

2. ***Why is each medication prescribed for this patient?***
3. ***Is each medication safe to administer to this patient?***
4. ***What assessment data would the nurse use to determine which pain medication to administer to this patient?***

Nurse Report

Victoria Smith is a female whose DOB is 10/03/1961, who is second post-op day for a right mastectomy. She is alert and oriented, heart rate is regular, and lungs have crackles in the bases. Pulse oximetry when awake is 95% on room air, but she drops to 87% while asleep, so she has had O_2 on 2 L last night. She received pain med X 2 last shift. She is up ad lib in the room. She is doing her incentive spirometry to 1500. Her right chest dressing is coming loose. Her JP drain has been putting out about 40 mL per shift. She is tolerating a regular diet. Her IV came out during the night, and I called and got an order to switch it to a saline lock. She refuses to look at the wound.

S Breast cancer
B Diagnosed with right breast adenocarcinoma, positive family history for breast cancer. Now **s/p** mastectomy
A Incision is 12 **cm** long, approximated, slightly red, dry and intact; JP draining 40 **mL** of serosanguinous fluid per shift
R Change dressing q shift and **PRN**, start saline lock, assess and treat pain as ordered

S Oxygen desaturation at night
B 15 pack-year smoking history. **SpO_2** ~95% in room air when awake, 87% when asleep.
A Desaturation related to splinting after surgery, pain meds and/or atelectasis
R Encourage deep breathing, **IS**, with 2 L **O_2** prn.

Additional Information

Married, 1 child.
Drinks alcohol occasionally
15 pack-year **Hx** of smoking
Has not been tested for BRCA-1 or BRCA-2 mutations. Hx of maternal grandmother with breast cancer.

? **Clinical Competency**

5. ***What is the primary problem for this patient?***
6. ***What are your priority assessments for this patient?***
7. ***What would you do first for this patient?***
8. ***What measures does the nurse take to protect the safety of the mastectomy operative side?***

References:

American Cancer Society (2010). Breast cancer. Retrieved August 1, 2010 from http://www.cancer.org/Cancer/BreastCancer/DetailedGuide/breast-cancer-risk-factors.
Deglin, J.H., Vallerand, A.H., & Sanoski, C.A. (2010). *Davis's Drug Guide for Nurses* (12th ed). F.A. Davis Company: Philadelphia, PA.
Venes, D. (Ed.). (2009). *Taber's Cyclopedic Medical Dictionary* (21st ed.). Philadelphia, PA: F.A. Davis Company.
Wilkinson, J.M. & Leuven K.V. (2007). *Fundamentals of Nursing: Theory, Concepts, & Applications.* Philadelphia, PA: F.A. Davis Co.
Williams, L.S. & Hopper, P.D. (2007). *Understanding Medical-Surgical Nursing* (3rd ed). Philadelphia, PA: F.A. Davis Co.

Cerebral Vascular Accident
Student Information

Introduction

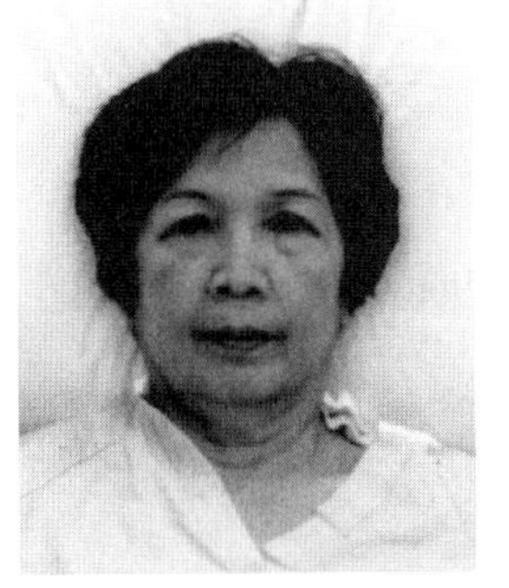

This simulation presents a female patient, whose DOB is 02/12/1947, admitted with symptoms of a **cerebral vascular accident (CVA)**, or stroke. She is experiencing right sided **hemiparesis** and **hyperglycemia**. The participants will manage the patient's signs and symptoms based on assessment findings.

Physiologic Concept

Oxygenation, Perfusion, Elimination, Mobility, Nutrition

Medical Diagnosis

CVA or "brain attack" occurs when a blood clot blocks an artery or a blood vessel breaks, interrupting blood flow to an area of the brain. When either of these happens, brain cells begin to die and brain damage occurs. Depending on where brain cells die during a stroke, abilities such as speech, movement and memory are affected.

There are two kinds of stroke. **Ischemic strokes** are more common and are caused by a blood clot that blocks a blood vessel in the brain. A **hemorrhagic stroke** is caused by a blood vessel that breaks and bleeds into the brain. It can also be caused by leakage from small intracerebral arteries damaged by chronic hypertension. "Mini-strokes" or **transient ischemic attacks (TIAs)** occur when the blood supply to the brain is briefly interrupted.

Controllable risk factors for CVA include high blood pressure, atrial fibrillation, high cholesterol, diabetes, atherosclerosis, smoking, obesity, drug abuse, and inactivity. Uncontrollable factors include age (over age 55), gender (male), being African American, Hispanic or Asian/Pacific Islander, or having a family history of stroke or transient ischemic attack (TIA).

Symptoms of stroke include:

- Sudden numbness or weakness of the face, arm or leg (especially on one side of the body)
- Sudden confusion, trouble speaking or understanding speech
- Sudden trouble seeing in one or both eyes
- Sudden trouble walking, dizziness, loss of balance or coordination
- Sudden severe headache with no known cause

Medications: Ischemic stroke can be treated with tissue plasminogen activator (t-PA) within a 4.5 hour window of initial symptoms. Other treatments include aspirin or other blood thinners, treatment for high blood pressure, high cholesterol, heart problems, or diabetes. Treatment for hemorrhagic stroke focuses on controlling bleeding and reducing pressure in the brain. If blood thinners were being taken, blood product transfusions may be needed to counter the effects of these medications.
Complications of a CVA include increased intracranial pressure and herniation, paralysis or loss of muscle movement, difficulty talking or

swallowing, memory loss or trouble with understanding, pain in parts of the body affected by the stroke, and changes in behavior and self-care.

An interdisciplinary rehabilitation plan following CVA includes physicians, nurses, dietician, physical therapist, occupational therapist, speech therapist, social worker and pastoral care as needed.

Learning Objectives

- ✓ Perform a complete assessment
- ✓ Recognize the signs & symptoms of a stroke
- ✓ Recognize the communication and mobility issues that occur due to a stroke depending on the area of the brain that is involved
- ✓ Care for patients with immobility issues and decrease effects on:
  - a) Skin
  - b) Joints and muscles (contractures)
  - c) Cardiovascular system
  - d) Urinary tract
  - e) Bowel elimination
- ✓ Assess need for assistance with ADLs
- ✓ Collaborate with other health professionals:
  - a) Physical therapist
  - b) Occupational therapist
  - c) Speech therapist
  - d) Social worker
  - e) Physician
  - f) Respiratory therapy
  - g) Unlicensed assistive personnel
- ✓ Identify safety factors for the post-CVA patient
- ✓ Identify CVA risk factors

Simulation Setting

Adult Patient Medical Unit

Participant Preparation

Knowledge Preparation:

- Review the pathophysiology and clinical manifestations of a right and left-sided CVA
- Review assessment needed for a patient with neurological deficit
- Review laboratory and diagnostic findings related to the patient who has had a CVA
- Review common treatments prescribed post-CVA
- Review safe oxygen delivery methods

Skill Preparation:

- Assessment, with a focus on respiratory, cardiovascular, and neurologic systems
- Application of oxygen delivery systems
- Intravenous site care
- Care for a patient with hemiparesis
- Medication administration

Evidence-Based Practice Recommendations

1. Immediate assessment for the patient experiencing a stroke should focus on the ABCs, with any compromise addressed. Additional assessment can include measurement of blood pressure, serum blood glucose, and neurological status, and obtaining a CT or MRI scan to assess injury. Admission is to a unit that can provide cardiac monitoring and management of seizures if needed.

2. Nursing interventions include monitoring of blood pressure and other vital signs, elevate head of bed up to maximum 30° with head midline, and administer medications as prescribed to control bleeding, pain and blood pressure. Initiate an intravenous access and obtain serum blood glucose.

3. Education focuses on medication teaching and rehabilitation training.

4. Health promotion includes support to return to the maximum level of functioning possible. Special care should be taken to prevent or manage skin breakdown, behavior changes, contractures, seizures, and depression.

Are You Ready?

1. What initial assessments would be performed for a patient suspected of having a stroke?

2. How would you perform a focused neurovascular assessment?

3. What are interventions to prevent complications after a stroke?

4. What do you expect to see in a patient who has experienced a right-sided versus a left-sided stroke?

5. Who are members of the interdisciplinary team that manage care for a stroke patient?

Continue on to meet the patient!

Cerebral Vascular Accident

Patient Information

Name	Medical Record Number	Birth Date	Allergies
Hettie Lee	869-24-745	02/12/1947	PCN, peanuts

Height	Weight	Gender	Attending Physician
62 inches	250 lbs	Female	Dr. Han Lee

Past Medical History

Hx of chronic **HA**;
Current home medications of 1 multivitamin daily

Initial Vital Signs on Admission

T 100.1°F, P 90, R 18, B/P 210/126, **SpO_2** 94% on RA
Headache pain 6/10

? Clinical Competency

1. ***What is your interpretation of the patient's vital signs?***

Physician Orders

Admit to monitor unit with hemiparesis r/t acute hemorrhagic stroke
Oxygen up to 4L per NC PRN to keep SpO_2 > 92%
VS q 2 hrs with pulse oximetry, neuro checks
Bed rest with Fall Precautions
NPO
Dulcolax (biscodyl) supp q 3 days if no BM
Normal Saline 100 mL/hr IV
Ativan (lorazepam) 1 mg IV q 15 min X 2 prn seizure activity and notify MD
Apply antiembolism stockings
TCDB q 2 hrs
Place foley cath
I/O
PT consult in am
OT consult in am
Social services consult for possible discharge placement
Speech therapy to evaluate swallowing
CXR, Chem 7, Chem 15, CBC, UA, ABG

? Clinical Competency

2. ***Why is each medication prescribed for this patient?***
3. ***Is each medication safe to administer to this patient?***
4. ***What are concerns the nurse has related to the physiologic status for this patient?***

Nurse Report

Hettie Lee is a female whose DOB is 02/12/1947, admitted after being found unconscious at home yesterday. She was diagnosed with acute hemorrhagic stroke by **MRI** in **ED**. She has an **IV** of **NS** running at 100 mL/hr. She continues to experience headache, blurry vision, decreased hearing, and right-side hemiparesis. Her smile droops on the right side, and she still has a headache. Headache pain is 6/10. She is **NPO**, with slurred speech. Heart rate is regular; lungs have some crackles bilaterally in the bases. No seizure activity has been noted. She received Lasix 40 mg IV, platelets and vitamin K in the ED. Initial blood glucose was 189. She is now incontinent, so she needs a foley.

S Hemiparesis
B New stroke
A Symptoms related to stroke, early in disease at risk for worsening. Initial B/P 210/126–received furosemide 40 mg IV in ED
R Evaluate extent of neurologic impairment, observe for stroke progression

S Hyperglycemia with capillary blood glucose of 189 in ED
B Noted on admission, no hx of diabetes.
A Likely related to stress response from acute stroke
R Review labs, recheck blood glucose as indicated

S Falls risk
B Did ambulate independently but now with acute stroke and weakness and vision/hearing change
A Fall risk r/t neurologic impairment from stroke
R Implement falls precautions

S Choking and aspiration risk
B New stroke, risk of airway motor impairment, slurred speech
A New aspiration risk, may be evolving
R Implement NPO status, observe for new or worsening symptoms

Additional Information

15 pack-year hx of smoking, quit 2 months ago, drinks occasional alcohol
Family hx of paternal hyperlipidemia and hyperglycemia, maternal hx of hypertension, maternal aunt hx of stroke

? **Clinical Competency**

*5. **What is the primary problem for this patient?***
*6. **What are your priority assessments for this patient?***
*7. **What would you do first for this patient?***

References

Deglin, J.H., Vallerand, A.H., & Sanoski, C.A. (2010). *Davis's Drug Guide for Nurses* (12th ed). F.A. Davis Company: Philadelphia, PA.

Mitka, M. (2007). Hemorrhagic stroke guidelines issued. *Journal of the American Medical Association*, 297, 2573–2575.

Stroke (2010) U.S. National Library of Medicine, Bethesda, MD. Retrieved August 1, 2010 from http://www.nlm.nih.gov/medlineplus/stroke.html

Venes, D. (Ed.). (2009). *Taber's Cyclopedic Medical Dictionary* (21st ed). Philadelphia, PA: F.A. Davis Company.

Wilkinson, J.M. & Leuven K.V. (2007). *Fundamentals of Nursing: Theory, Concepts, & Applications.* Philadelphia, PA: F.A. Davis Co.

Williams, L.S. & Hopper, P.D. (2007). *Understanding Medical-Surgical Nursing* (3rd ed). Philadelphia, PA: F.A. Davis Co. Davis Co.

Sickle Cell Anemia
Student Information

Introduction

This simulation presents an African American patient whose DOB is 02/12/1980, in **Sickle Cell Crisis**. Despite treatment the patient has ongoing pain, fatigue, and **hypoxia**. The participants will manage the patient's signs and symptoms based on assessment findings.

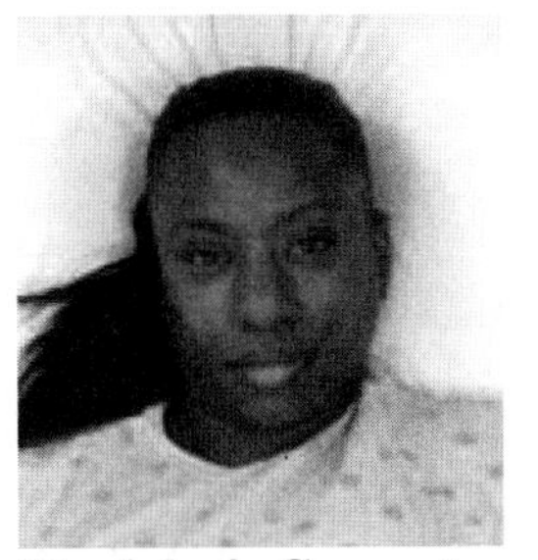

Physiologic Concept

Oxygenation, Circulatory, Hematologic

Medical Diagnosis

Sickle Cell Anemia is a **hemolytic anemia** that results from the inheritance of the sickle hemoglobin gene. This gene causes an abnormal form of hemoglobin in the **erythrocyte**. A crystal-like formation of the **hemoglobin** occurs when it is exposed to low oxygen levels. When erythrocytes experience conditions that result in decreased oxygen levels, they become stiff and sickle shaped. The blood flow can become obstructed because the sickled cells clump together. This obstruction can lead to **ischemia** and **infarction** of the surrounding tissue. When normal oxygen levels are restored, the sickled erythrocyte can resume their normal shape. Frequent episodes of **sickling** and unsickling can contribute to a weakening of the erythrocyte cell membranes.

Sickle Cell Anemia is often diagnosed during infancy or early childhood. Many people with this disease will die as middle aged adults from pulmonary and renal failure. Clinical manifestations seen with this disorder consist of anemia, **pallor**, fatigue, and pain. Chronic hypoxia can lead to organ and tissue damage. Many people will experience Sickle Cell Crisis which results from tissue hypoxia and necrosis. The Sickle Cell Crisis can hasten tissue hypoxia and acidic metabolic waste products. This can contribute to additional sickling and cell damage.

Nursing care is directed toward alleviating symptoms, complications, and organ damage. Treatment usually consists of medications, oxygen, blood transfusions, hydration therapy, and pain management.

Learning Objectives

- ✓ Identify and check the symptoms of Sickle Cell Anemia
- ✓ Complete a thorough pain assessment
  - a) Administer analgesics
  - b) Incorporate complementary therapy
- ✓ Utilize therapeutic communication techniques
- ✓ Perform pulse oximetry measurement
- ✓ Administer oxygen
- ✓ Document all aspects of patient care

Simulation Setting

Adult Patient Medical Unit

Participant Preparation

Knowledge Preparation:

- Review the pathophysiology and clinical manifestations of Sickle Cell Anemia
- Review assessment needed for a patient with Sickle Cell Anemia
- Review oxygen delivery methods for a patient with Sickle Cell Anemia
- Review laboratory and diagnostic findings related to tissue hypoxia for a patient with Sickle Cell Anemia
- Review pain management for a patient with Sickle Cell Anemia

Skill Preparation:

- Assessment of the cardiopulmonary and neurological systems
- Medication administration
- Application of oxygen delivery systems
- Measurement of oxygen saturation levels
- Pain assessment

Evidence-Based Practice Recommendations

1. All individuals identified as having Sickle Cell Crisis will be assessed appropriately. An assessment of all body systems must be conducted.
   Pain assessment should include:
   - Pain level
   - Intensity
   - Quality
   - Frequency
   - Aggravating and alleviating factors
   - Determine if current pain experienced is the same or different from the pain the patient usually experienced in a crisis

   Cardiopulmonary assesment should include:
   - Vital signs
   - Chest ausculation
   - Level of dyspnea
   - Prescence of tachycardia
   - Pulse oximetry
   - Prescence of peripheral edema
   - Mucuous membranes
   - Level of fatigue
   - Fluid intake/output
   - Urine output
   - Skin turgor

   Neurologic assessment should include:
   - Level of consciousness
   - Orientation

   Assess for the presence of infection in the:
   - Legs
   - Chest
   - Skin

2. Nurses will be able to implement interventions for Sickle Cell Crisis.
   - Controlled oxygen therapy
   - Monitor and manage pain
   - Medications
   - Prevent and manage infections
   - Energy conserving strategies
   - Relaxation techniques
   - Assist in establishing priorities in performing tasks or activities
   - Assist in developing a schedule of activities that allows for alteration of exercise and rest periods
   - Manage potential complications

3. Patient education will be provided to increase the knowledge of the disease.
   - Assist to understand disease process
   - Self care techniques to decrease oxygen consumption
   - Provide information on situations that can precipitate a crisis
   - Increase knowledge of all medications

4. Health promotion will be encouraged by providing information regarding consequences and characteristics of Sickle Cell Disease and teaching activities that can maintain wellness.
   - Avoid infections
   - Adequate hydration
   - Avoid exposure to cold temperatures
   - Stress reduction activities
   - Avoid overexertion
   - Avoid smoking
   - Develop coping skills
   - Avoid high altitudes
   - Adequeate rest and sleep

Are You Ready?

1. What behavioral responses should the nurse assess for when a patient has pain?
2. What pain management techniques can be used to promote comfort?
3. When would the nurse reassess the patient's pain level?
4. What are manifestations of pain?
5. What personal experiences of the patient affect their pain?
6. What nursing interventions can the nurse implement to increase oxygenation?

Continue on to meet the patient!

Patient Information

Name	Medical Record Number	Birth Date	Allergies
Shanay Thomas	928-64-492	02/12/1980	NKDA Allergic to pollen and ragweed

Height	Weight	Gender	Attending Physician
65 in	135 lbs	Female	Dr. Han Lee

Past Medical History

This patient was diagnosed with **Sickle Cell Anemia** at 8 years old. Previous hospitalizations with Sickle Cell Crisis.

Initial Vital Signs

T 99.4°F, P 96, R 26, B/P 116/72, Pain 9/10, O_2 sat 90%

? Clinical Competency

1. ***What is your interpretation of the vital signs?***

Physician Orders

Oxygen O_2 2**L**/min per **NC**; titrate to keep O_2 sat > 94% min
Hydroxyurea (hydrea) 1000 **mg po** daily
Folic Acid (folvite) 1 mg po **qd**
Colace (docusate sodium) 100 mg po **bid**
Motrin (ibuprofen) 600 mg **q6h**
Ferrous sulfate 325 mg po qd
Morphine sulfate 10–15 mg **IV,** every 3–4 hours prn for pain
Toradol (ketorolac) 15 mg IM q6h prn for pain
Tylenol (acetaminophen) 650 mg po, every 4–6 hours prn for temperature elevation greater than 100.4 °F.
IV, D5 0.9% NaCl@ 60 mL
Vital signs **q4h**
Regular diet
Bedrest

? Clinical Competency

2. ***Why has this patient been placed on bed rest?***
3. ***Is each medication safe to administer to this patient?***
4. ***What should you consider to determine which prn medication is appropriate for this patient?***

Nurse Report

Shanay Thomas is a female whose DOB is 02/12/1980, admitted 4 days ago in Sickle Cell Crisis. She has been experiencing severe pain in her chest, back, arms, and legs despite treatment. Her breathing is regular and non-labored and she experiences SOB on exertion. She is anxious, irritable, and frustrated as a result of her discomfort. On admission the SpO_2 was 90%. Oxygen is being administered at 2L per NC with a current SpO_2 of 88%.

S Pain 9/10
B Received morphine sulfate 10 mg 3 hours ago, still c/o pain
A Evaluate effectiveness of current pain medication
R Assess and treat pain as ordered, consider dosage adjustment. Provide complimentary pain relief therapies.

S Persistent hypoxia despite NC oxygen
B Sickle Cell Crisis
A Monitor pulse oximetry and symptoms of hypoxia
R Titrate oxygen therapy to maintain SpO2 >94% as ordered
Position for comfort and maximum gas exchange

Additional Information

Ms. Miles is single and does not have children.
Family history: Aunt with Sickle Cell Disease
Occasional social drinker

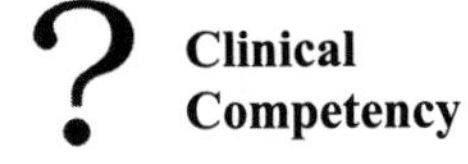

Clinical Competency

5. ***What is your primary problem for this patient?***
6. ***What are your priority assessments for this patient?***

References

National Heart, Lung, and Blood Institute: National Institute of Health (2004). The management of sickle cell disease. U.S. Department of Health & Human Services: Rockville, MD.

Deglin, J.H., Vallerand, A.H., & Sanoski, C.A. (2010). *Davis's Drug Guide for Nurses* (12th ed). F.A. Davis Company: Philadelphia, PA.

Venes, D. (Ed.). (2009). *Taber's Cyclopedic Medical Dictionary* (21st ed.). Philadelphia, PA: F.A. Davis Company.

Wilkinson, J.M. & Leuven K.V. (2007). *Fundamentals of Nursing: Theory, Concepts, & Applications.* Philadelphia, PA: F.A. Davis Co.

Williams, L.S. & Hopper, P.D. (2007). *Understanding Medical-Surgical Nursing* (3rd ed). Philadelphia, PA: F.A. Davis Co.

Chronic Kidney Disease
Student Information

Introduction

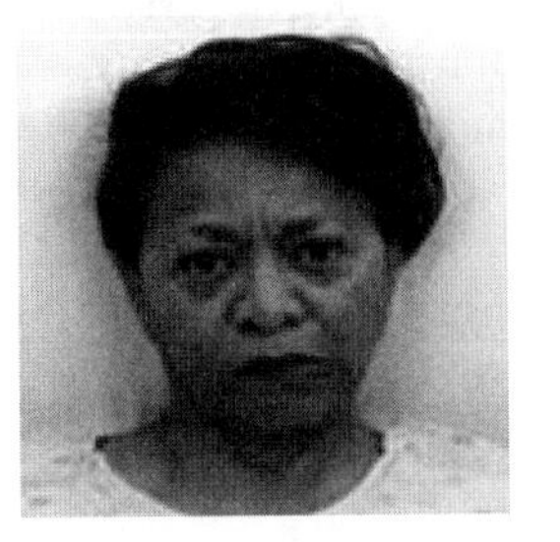

This simulation presents an African American female whose DOB is 08/09/1942, with a history of **Stage 4 Chronic Kidney Disease.** She was admitted for **Chronic Renal Failure (CRF)** and the surgical creation of an **AV fistula.** The patient presents with anemia, fatigue, shortness of breath (**SOB**) with activity. The participants will manage the signs and symptoms based on assessment findings.

Physiologic Concept

Elimination, Fluid and Electrolytes

Medical Diagnosis

Chronic Kidney Disease (CKD) occurs when a person has a decreased kidney function over an extended period of time. This decline in kidney function is irreversible and last for 3 or more months. When the kidney function has deteriorated to the point that renal dialysis is needed, the patient will progress to the final stage of CKD. The final stage will also develop if CKD is untreated and is often referred to as Chronic Renal Failure (CRF) or **End Stage Renal Disease (ESRD).**

With the loss of kidney function, the kidneys will be unable to excrete metabolic waste. They will also develop difficulty regulating fluid and electrolyte balance. The end products of metabolism will build up in the blood as kidney function decreases. As a result, uremia will develop and negatively impact every body system. The rate of decline in kidney function can range from months to years and is dependent upon the underlying disorder. Many patients will experience an increase in health care needs, diminished quality of life, and premature death.

Hypertension, diabetes, obesity, and cardiovascular diseases increase the risk of developing CKD. African Americans and Native Americans have an increased risk for developing CKD. Hypertension and diabetes are common in African Americans and Native Americans. Kidney function declines with aging. Elderly individuals have an increased risk of kidney dysfunction. Many elderly individuals also have other diseases that can increase the risk for developing CKD.

There is no cure for CKD. Treatment is focused on slowing the progression, managing underlying causes or conditions, replacing the loss of kidney function, and preventing complications of the disease.

Learning Objectives

- ✓ Recognize stages of chronic kidney disease
- ✓ Educate the patient regarding food and fluid restrictions
- ✓ Correlate pathophysiology of disease to assessment findings
- ✓ Identify complications related to end stage renal disease (ESRD) or chronic renal failure (CRF)

Simulation Setting

Adult Patient Medical Unit

Participant Preparation

Knowledge Preparation:

- Review the pathophysiology and clinical manifestations of CRF
- Review assessment needed for the patient with a CRF
- Review the procedure for administering and maintaining IV fluids
- Review laboratory and diagnostic findings for a CRF
- Review how to prepare the patient for surgery

Skill Preparation:

- Assessment with a focus on the neurological, cardiovascular, pulmonary, gastrointestinal, integumentary, hematological, reproductive, musculoskeletal system
- Medication administration
- Assess **IV** site and flush saline lock

Evidence-Based Practice Recommendations

1. All individuals identified as having a CRF will be assessed appropriately. The nurse should obtain vital signs, conduct an assessment on the neurological, cardiovascular, pulmonary, gastrointestinal, integumentary, hematological, reproductive, and musculoskeletal system. The diagnostic laboratory results must be monitored.

2. Nurses will be able to implement appropriate interventions for CRF. Nursing interventions should include monitoring all laboratory and diagnostic results, kidney function, weight, fluid and electroylyte imbalances, elimination pattern, assessment of dietary habits, maintain nutrition, and if needed, prepare the patient for surgery.

7. Education for the patient with CRF should include information on the disease process, hypertension, anemia, diet, exercise programs, and medications.

8. Health promotion includes the importance of monitoring blood pressure, reduction in alcohol and salt intake, and maintaining follow-up appointments. The patient should be informed to have immunizations to prevent illness, report changes in the appearance and volume of urine, and frequency of urination.

Are You Ready?

1. What would you expect a patient to look like who is experiecing a CRF?

2. What signs and symptoms would the nurse assess for in a patient with CRF?

3. What questions would you ask the patient regarding their urinary elimination pattern?

4. What are your priority nursing interventions for a patient with a CRF?

Continue on to meet the patient!

Patient Information

Name	Medical Record Number	Birth Date	Allergies
Charlene Miles	100-34-756	08/09/1942	NKDA Seasonal Allergies

Height	Weight	Gender	Attending Physician
70 in	170 lbs	Female	Dr. Han Lee

Past Medical History

Chronic Kidney Disease
End Stage Renal Disease
Hypertension

Initial Vital Signs

Vital signs: T 100.1°F, P 98, R 20, BP142/84, SpO2 95% RA, Pain 0/10

? Clinical Competency

1. ***What is your interpretation of the vital signs?***
2. ***What is a precipitating factor that could have contributed to the development of Ms. Miles CRF?***

Physician Orders

Oxygen 2 L via nasal cannula for O_2 sat < 93%
Lopressor (metoprolol) 100**mg po bid**
Nifedipine (procardia) 10mg po **tid**
Lasix (furosemide) 60mg po tid
Epoetin (erythropoietin) 4000 units subcut
Tylenol (acetaminophen) 650mg po q-4–6h prn pain
Saline lock
Saline flush **q** shift
Bedrest
VSq4h
NPO

? Clinical Competency

3. ***Why is each medication prescribed for this patient?***
4. ***How does renal failure affect the metabolism of medications?***

Nurse Report

Charlene Miles is a female whose DOB is 08/09/1942, admitted with Chronic Renal Failure. She is scheduled to have an AV fistula inserted because the frequency of her dialysis must be increased. Assessment reveals she is awake, alert, oriented X3. Breathing is regular and non-labored. Lungs are clear bilaterally. She has complaints of feeling tired and weak. Ms. Miles states she is able to urinate in very small amount amounts.

S Complains of fatigue
B History of CKD
Elective admission for **Arteriovenous (AV) fistula** creation
A Weak and tired most likely from anemia
R Assess patient and assist her with care. Follow up with labs

Additional Information

Single, no children
Cigarettes: None.
Alcohol: Denies alcohol intake
Possible paternal DM

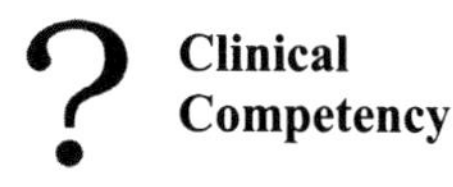

5. What is your primary problem for this patient?

References

Agency for Healthcare Research and Quality (2008). Chronic kidney disease—identification, evaluation and management of patients. U.S. Department of Health & Human Services: Rockville, MD.

Agency for Healthcare Research and Quality (2007). KDOQI clinical practice guidelines and clinical practice recommendations for anemia in chronic kidney disease: update of hemoglobin target. U.S. Department of Health & Human Services: Rockville, MD.

Deglin, J.H., Vallerand, A.H., & Sanoski, C.A. (2010). *Davis's Drug Guide for Nurses* (12th ed). F.A. Davis Company: Philadelphia, PA.

Venes, D. (Ed.). (2009). *Taber's Cyclopedic Medical Dictionary* (21st ed.). Philadelphia, PA: F.A. Davis Company.

Wilkinson, J.M. & Leuven K.V. (2007). *Fundamentals of Nursing: Theory, Concepts, & Applications.* Philadelphia, PA: F.A. Davis Co.

Williams, L.S. & Hopper, P.D. (2007). *Understanding Medical-Surgical Nursing* (3rd ed). Philadelphia, PA: F.A. Davis Co.

Appendix A

Clinical Competency Discussions

Simulation 1: Chronic Obstructive Pulmonary Disease

1. What is your interpretation of the patient's vital signs?

The admission VS were: T 98.4°F- P 88- R 20- B/P 126/84- SpO2 93% RA
These values are WNL, but frequent monitoring is needed as the patient status, especially the respiratory status, can change quickly. Note that the patient has reported increasing SOB, which can be an early sign of an underlying status change.

2. Why is each medication prescribed for this patient?

Prednisolone 80 mg—a corticosteroid to suppress inflammation in chronic illnesses such as COPD.
Aspirin 81 mg—at this dose is used as prophylaxis for MI. A patient with COPD is at greater risk for MI. Should not be used with alcohol. Remember Mr. Winston already has had one MI.
Atrovent (ipratropium bromide) MDI 2 puffs—used to produce bronchodilation in the COPD patient. The inhaled route reduces systemic anticholinergic effects. Not for quick relief of bronchospasm.
Albuterol MDI 2 puffs prn—used for quick-relief agent to relieve bronchospasm. Used in addition to the Atrovent during COPD exacerbation for bronchdilation.
Lasix (furosemide) 40 mg—used to decrease excess fluid to decrease edema and lower blood pressure. The patient's B/P is WNL, and nursing assessment will evaluate for edema. Potassium level should be monitored.
Lopressor (metoprolol) 50 mg—a beta-blocker used to treat hypertension, especially in those like Mr. Winston who have had a MI. Note that the B/P is WNL.
Lanoxin (digoxin) 0.125 mg—increases myocardial contraction leading to increased cardiac output and slowing of the heart rate. Note that the apical pulse MUST be assessed prior to administration, and the elderly are at greater risk for toxicity. With the patient's history of MI and heart failure, this medication should help the heart function.

3. Is each medication safe to administer to this patient?

The prednisolone dose is higher than the 60 mg/day recommended for most uses. The dose may need clarified with the care provider.
Aspirin prescribed at this dose is appropriate to decrease platelet aggregation to lower MI risk.
The other prescribed medications are safe to administer as prescribed.

4. What are concerns the nurse has with administering oxygen at a high rate to this patient?

High rates of oxygen administration may decrease the drive to breathe in the patient with COPD and even make them stop breathing spontaneously. A low arterial oxygen level is this patient's primary drive for breathing. Oxygen needs are determined by oxygen saturation by pulse oximetry and also ABG results. The patient should be monitored closely once oxygen is started for signs of drowsiness or other changes in level of consciousness, indicating that the patient is in distress.

5. What is the primary problem for this patient?

The deteriorating respiratory status is the primary problem. With the history of COPD, MI, HTN, and heart failure, this patient may quickly develop respiratory distress.

6. What are your priority assessments for this patient?

A respiratory assessment will monitor the amount of distress the patient is experiencing, and the need for additional interventions. The cardiac system is very sensitive to oxygen levels, and with the patient history of heart failure and MI, a thorough assessment that includes checking for pain and signs of heart failure is important. Level of consciousness is an indicator of oxygenation for the patient.

7. What would you do first for this patient?

Interventions to address the decreasing oxygenation of the patient should be initiated: raise the head of the bed to a semi-Fowler's or Fowler's position, apply oxygen at low levels to increase oxygenation saturation, encourage pursed lip breathing to decrease air-trapping, assess respiratory status, assess orientation, and continue to monitor the patient status. Review the ABG results and other diagnostics to ascertain if additional interventions are needed. Assess the need for prn medications to improve breathing.

Simulation 2: Hip Fracture

1. What is your interpretation of the vital signs? T 100.0°F, P 90, R 20, BP120/95, SpO2 95% RA, Pain 6/10

The temperature is elevated. It must be monitored. An elevated temperature could be a sign of infection. The pulse, respirations, and SpO2 are WNL. The blood pressure is elevated. The patient does have a history of hypertension. Determine the baseline blood pressure and when the patient received the last dose of hypertensive medication. The patient is experiencing pain. This could also contribute to the blood pressure elevating. Conduct a pain assessment and give pain medication as ordered.

2. What circulatory responses should the nurses assess for when a patient has a hip fracture?

The nurse should assess the affected leg for color. A pink color would be a normal finding. A pale color could indicate decreased circulating oxygen and blood. Venous congestion could be seen as cyanosis. The dorsalis pedis and posterior tibial pulses should be assessed evaluate arterial blood flow. Capillary refill, temperature, edema, helps provide information regarding perfusion. Pain that is not relieved with medication could indicate neurovascular problem.

3. Why is each medication prescribed for this patient?

Morphine Sulfate 2 mg—An opioid analgesic used to treat moderate to severe pain.
Zocor (simvastatin) Zocor 40 mg—increases level of good cholesterol (HDL) and decreases levels of bad cholesterol (LDL). It is given to decrease the cholesterol level. The patient has a history of hyperlipidemia.
Micardis (telmisartan) 12.5 mg—inhibits vasoconstriction and aldosterone which work to lower the blood pressure. The patient has hypertension.
Tylenol (acetaminophen) 650 mg—produces analgesia and decreases body temperature. It is used to relieve mild to moderate pain and decrease fever.
Lovenox (enoxaparin) 30 mg—A low molecular weight Heparin that is administered to prevent clot formation.

4. Is each medication safe to administer to this patient?

Yes each medication is safe to administer.

5. What is your primary problem for this patient?

The postoperative hip fracture patient will often have complaints of severe pain. Regular assessment of pain should be conducted. The pain assessment should include the location, duration, pain scale, aggravating and alleviating factors, and quality of the pain. Medications should be given as ordered to adequately manage the pain. Movement can be very painful. This could make the person avoid moving and contribute to immobility. The longer a person is immobile the greater the risk for complications such as deep vein thrombosis, pneumonia, and pressure ulcers.

Simulation 3: Dementia

1. What is your interpretation of the patient's vital signs?

Initial vital signs are reported as T 99°F, P 68, R 16, B/P 114/68, SpO2 95% on RA, pain 0/10. These vital signs are WNL for this patient.

2. Why is each medication prescribed for this patient?

Donepezil (Aricept) 10 mg po—slows the breakdown of acetylcholine, which is needed to form memories.
Memantine (Namenda) 10mg po—expected outcome is to improve learning and memory.
Multi-vitamin 1 po—used to meet nutritional needs for a patient who may not eat regularly.
Docusate (Colace) 100 mg po—used to soften stools. Appropriate for a patient who has limited mobility and irregular eating habits.
Synthroid (Levothyroxine sodium) 0.1 mg po—thyroid supplement. The patient has a history of hypothyroidism.

3. Is each medication safe to administer to this patient?

Each medication is appropriate and safe for this patient.

4. What medication administration problems may arise in a patient who is confused?

A confused patient may not understand the need, or understand the request to take medications. Incorporating medication administration into a regular routine may enhance compliance. Carefully consider the ethics of "hiding" medications in food when determining administration techniques.

5. What is the primary problem for this patient?

Safety is the priority concern for this patient, followed by meeting ADL needs. Set up the room environment to protect the patient's safety and sense of security. Assist with ADLs as needed.

6. What are your priority assessments for this patient?

Mental status is the priority assessment for this patient in order to plan appropriate care and safety. Frustration and anxiety from being in a new environment can be exhibited with behavioral issues. Assessment for caregiver strain is also a priority for this family.

7. What would you do first for this patient?

An assessment is needed to evaluate the overall status of the patient, specifically looking or a change in mental status or physical status that would account for the increased confusion.

8. How can you meet the safety needs for this patient?

Bed alarms, top siderails raised, monitoring by staff/family, nightlight, decreased background noise, and limiting visitors can all address patient safety needs related to the environment. Monitoring fluid and food intake, elimination and sleep patterns can help address physiological safety needs.

Simulation 4: Heart Failure

1. What is your interpretation of the patient's vital signs?

The initial vital signs were: T 97.8°F , P 92, R 20, B/P 154/86, SpO_2 94% on room air, Pain 0/10
The initial VS indicate increased blood pressure, with additional VS stable with the report of increasing SOB noted which may require the use of supplemental oxygen. The patient has a hx of HTN, which is a major risk factor for heart failure.

2. Why is each medication prescribed for this patient?

Lasix (furosemide) 40 mg po—is needed to remove excess fluid and sodium that increases the work load of the heart.
Lanoxin (digoxin) 0.125 mg po—increases myocardial contraction leading to increased cardiac output and slowing of the heart rate. Note that the apical pulse MUST be assessed prior to administration, and the elderly are at greater risk for toxicity. With the patient's history of MI and heart failure, this medication should help the heart function.
Vasotec (enalapril) 10 mg po—an ACE inhibitor to expand blood vessels and decrease peripheral resistance to decrease the workload of the heart.
Lopressor (metoprolol) 50 mg po—a beta-blocker used to treat hypertension, especially in those like Mr. Winston who have had a MI. Note that the B/P is WNL.
Potassium chloride 20 mEq po—appropriate to supplement the potassium loss from the daily use of Lasix.

3. Is each medication safe to administer to this patient?

These doses are safe to administer to this patient.

4. How are signs and symptoms for right-sided heart failure different from left-sided heart failure?

Signs and symptoms of left-sided heart failure include: weakness, oliguria in day and nocturia at night, confusion, dizziness, pallor, weak peripheral pulses, cough worse at night, dyspnea, crackles or wheezes, pink/frothy sputum.

Signs and symptoms of right-sided heart failure include: JVD, enlarged liver/spleen, anorexia and nausea, dependent edema, distended abdomen, swollen hands and fingers, weight gain, polyuria at night, increased B/P from excess volume, or decreased B/P from failure.

Symptoms of worsening heart failure include rapid weight gain (3 lb in a week), decrease in activity tolerance over 2–3 days, cough lasting 3–5 days, nocturia, dyspnea especially at rest.

5. What is the primary problem for this patient?

Although this patient was admitted with a cardiac problem (heart failure), the primary problem comes from the respiratory status of the patient. Increasing SOB and decreasing pulse oximetry must be dealt with immediately (remember the A-B-Cs of prioritization). Stabilize the respiratory status, and then implement measures that will help the respiratory and cardiac systems, such as the administration of the diuretic. The IV route has a rapid onset of action, and can pull off excess fluid to assist in breathing and decrease the workload of the heart.

6. What are your priority assessments for this patient?

A respiratory assessment will evaluate the amount of distress the patient is experiencing and the need for additional interventions. The underlying disease process of heart failure places both the respiratory and cardiac systems at risk; a thorough cardiac assessment, including assessment for abdominal and peripheral edema, is very important. Mental status and electrolyte assessment also evaluates the function of the respiratory and cardiac systems.

7. What would you do first for this patient?

Interventions to address the decreasing oxygenation of the patient should be initiated: raise the head of the bed to a semi-Fowler's or Fowler's position, apply oxygen at low levels to increase oxygenation saturation, encourage pursed lip breathing to decrease air-trapping, assess respiratory status, assess orientation, and continue to monitor the patient status. Measures to improve cardiac function include the administration of the diuretic (which may need to be prescribed by IV route for faster effect) and other prescribed medications. Evaluate the effectiveness of medications administered. Limit activity until the cardiac status is more stable.

Simulation 5: Small Bowel Obstruction

1. ***What is your interpretation of the vital signs?*** T 97.8F, P 88, R 20, BP125/84, SpO2 94% RA, Pain 9/10

The admission vital signs are WNL. It is important to monitor the vital signs frequently because the patient status could change quickly. A pain level of 9 indicates severe pain. Many patients are often restless and changes positions frequently in an effort to decrease discomfort. A pain assessment should be performed and pain medication should be administered as ordered?

2. ***What factors made Mr. Bloch a risk for developing a bowel obstruction?***

Mr. Bloch has Crohn's disease. He has an extensive history of intestinal problems in the past. Recently he experienced a change in bowel habits which contributed to him not having a bowel movement in a couple of days. .

3. ***Why is each medication prescribed for this patient?***

Mesalamine (Apriso) 800mg—a anti-inflammatory medication that stops the body from producing a substance that can cause inflammation and pain.
Omeprazole (Prilosec) 20mg—A proton pump inhibitor that blocks acid that is produced in of in the stomach. It can be used in patients with acid-induced inflammation in the stomach and intestinal tract. Mr. Bloch has a history of Crohn's disease.
Hyoscyamine (Anaspaz) 0.25mg—This medication reduces the movement of the intestines and stomach and fluids in the stomach.
Morphine Sulfate 1.5 mg—An opioid analgesic used to treat moderate to severe pain.

4. ***Is each medication safe to administer to this patient?***

All medications are safe to administer.

5. ***What is your primary problem for this patient?***

The primary problem for this patient is bowel elimination. The intestinal obstruction must be relieved to prevent strangulation, necrosis, perforation, and peritonitis. Since this patient has been vomiting for 14 hours there is an increase risk for a fluid volume deficit.

6. ***What are your priority assessments for this patient?***

A gastrointestinal assessment is needed to monitor the amount of distress the patient is experiencing and how the disease is progressing. The nurse should assess VS, mouth, bowel sounds, abdominal girth, abdominal pain, nausea, vomiting, rectum, the passing of flatus and fecal material. It is also important for the patient to be assessed for dehydration. Additional assessments should include signs of electrolyte imbalances, fluid intake and output, and laboratory results.

Simulation 6: Diabetes Mellitus

1. What is your interpretation of the vital signs?

The admission VS were: T 97.8F, P 68, R 18, BP142/88, SpO2 99% RA, Pain 1/10.
The temperature, pulse, respirations and pulse oximetry are WNL, but frequent monitoring is needed. The blood pressure is elevated. There is a history of hypertension. It is important to determine normal blood pressure patterns for this patient. Review the MAR and talk to the patient to determine the last dose of hypertensive medication. Pain rated 1/10 is considered minimal discomfort. A pain assessment must be conducted.

2. Why is each medication prescribed for this patient?

Lantus insulin 20 units—is a long acting insulin used to enhance the passage of glucose across cell membranes, which will help to lower blood glucose levels over an extended period of time. This medication should be administered at the same time each day. The nurse must monitor blood glucose levels, food intake, and complications of diabetes.

Regular insulin (sliding scale)—a clear short acting insulin used to enhance the passage of glucose across cell membranes, which will help to lower blood glucose levels. It is usually administered before meals alone or in combination with longer acting insulin. It is the only insulin that can be administered intravenously. The nurse must monitor blood glucose levels, food intake, and complications of diabetes.

Valsartan (diovan) 80mg—is used to treat hypertension in this patient by blocking angiotensin II. As a result the blood vessels dilate and blood pressure is lowered. The nurse must monitor the blood pressure.

Potassium chloride 40 IV mEq—is used to treat hypokalemia. The patient's potassium level is low. Diabetic ketoacidosis can cause hypokalemia. The nurse must monitor the heart rate, rhythm, and potassium level.

Tylenol (acetaminophen) 325 mg produces analgesia and decreases body temperature. It is used to relieve mild to moderate pain and decrease fever.

3. Is each medication safe to administer to this patient?

All medications are safe to administer as prescribed.

4. What is your primary problem for this patient?

Diabetic ketoacidosis is the primary problem for this patient. This disorder often causes dehydration which can contribute to a low potassium level. It must be managed appropriately by treating the hyperglycemia, correcting the dehydration, and electrolyte imbalances.

5. What are your priority assessments for this patient?

Cardiopulmonary assessments are very important for this patient. There is a risk for a fluid and electrolyte imbalance and hyperventilation. The hyperglycemia will cause polydipsia and polyuria, which can contribute to the development of dehydration. In order to maintain tissue perfusion, rehydration is needed. The rehydration increases the risk for fluid overload and hypokalemia. The nurse must also monitor for symptoms of hypokalemia, VS, mental status changes, acetone breath, urinary output, and laboratory results.

6. What are symptoms of hypoglycemia and why is this patient at risk for developing this disorder?

Hypoglycemia occurs when the blood glucose levels fall below 60 mg/dL. Some of the symptoms that result from hypoglycemia consist of sweating, tremors, nausea, hunger, anxiety, irritability, hypotension, headache, and blurred vision. Insulin is given to manage diabetic ketoacidosis. The insulin works to lower the blood glucose levels. If the blood glucose levels decrease too much, the patient will develop hypoglycemia.

Simulation 7: Post-Operative Care Post-Mastectomy

1. What is your interpretation of the patient's vital signs?

Initial vital signs are T 101.7°F, P 88, R 20, B/P 126/84, SpO2 95% on RA pain 3/10.
The increase in temperature is likely due to an inflammatory process related to surgery, but wound assessment for infection is important. The pulse rate may be affected by the current pain level of the patient. The pulse ox level is normal, but lower than might be expected in an otherwise healthy adult; respiratory assessment is important.

2. Why is each medication prescribed for this patient?

Morphine sulfate 2 mg IV Q 2 hours prn—administered for moderate to severe pain. Has rapid onset but a shorter half-life than other routes. Note respiratory side effects.
Tylenol (acetaminophen) 650mg po Q 4 hours prn—anti-inflammatory medication that relieves mild to moderate pain. This medication can be given when oral intake is being tolerated well.
MVI (multivitamin) 1 tab po daily—multivitamin dietary supplement to improve nutritional status.
FeSO4 (ferrous sulfate) 1 tab po daily—iron sulfate dietary supplement used to improve anemia status, hemoglobin status.

3. Is each medication safe to administer to this patient?

These medications are safe to administer, although the choice of pain medication is dependent on nursing judgment and patient status.

4. What assessment data would the nurse use to determine which pain medication to administer to a patient?

Factors such as level of pain, oral intake status, break through pain, level of pain, patient preference, and previous success with pain management are all factors to consider.

5. What is the primary problem for this patient?

The immediate problem for this patient is pain management. The saline lock may need to be started to give pain med.

6. What are your priority assessments for this patient?

Priority assessments include pain assessment and emotional status. Wound/drain assessment is also important due to the reported temperature.

7. What would you do first for this patient?

After assessment to determine baseline status, pain medication would be administered. Additional interventions include restarting the saline lock (may be needed to administer pain medication selected), deep breathing with IS due to desaturation when sleeping. Once patient comfort is established, emotional issues can be addressed.

8. What measures does the nurse take to protect the safety of the mastectomy operative side?

There is a risk of lymphedema post-mastectomy. To decrease this risk, the operative side should be used for IV access, and blood pressure should be measured on the opposite extremity. Physical therapy is often prescribed to improve range of motion on the operative side, especially is the surgery is extensive.

Simulation 8: Cerebral Vascular Accident

1. What is your interpretation of the patient's vital signs?

Initial vital signs were: T 100.1°F, P 90, R 18, B/P 210/126, $SpO2_{94}$% on RA, headache pain 4/10. The temperature and blood pressure are notably increased. This may be indicative of intracerebral pressure. While blood pressure can be increased related to pain, the level of increase is more likely linked to the underlying dynamics of the hemorrhagic stroke. Headache pain can also occur with the increased blood pressure. The health care provider should be notified of the blood pressure.

2. Why is each medication prescribed for this patient?

Normal Saline 100 mL/hr IV—an isotonic solution is indicated for post-stroke fluid balance needs.

Ativan (lorazepam) 1 mg IV prn seizure activity—seizure activity needs to be treated emergently to decrease intracranial pressure and limit additional damage.

Dulcolax (biscodyl) supp q 3 days—constipation is the most common bowel problem after a stroke. Use of a suppository can help maintain regular bowel function. Note that a vaso-vagal response with suppository use may cause a decrease in heart rate.

Note that there is nothing for pain ordered.

3. Is each medication safe to administer to this patient?

Administering a suppository can increase intracranial pressure-assess other s/s first. Other prescribed medications are safe.

4. What are concerns the nurse has related to the physiologic status for this patient?

Airway, breathing, and circulation are critical concerns for this patient, including aspiration risk. Additionally, the neurological status and blood pressure need close monitoring. Temperature, hyperglycemia and high blood pressure need to be managed.

5. What is the primary problem for this patient?

Stabilization of the patient's airway is critical. Monitoring neurological and cardiac status is indicative of overall function of the brain. Keep NPO and monitor respiratory, neurologic and cardiac status.

6. *What are your priority assessments for this patient?*

Respiratory assessment is the priority assessment. Supplemental oxygen may be needed not only due to oxygen saturation, but respiratory failure can occur from increased intracranial pressure or if the brainstem is involved. Keep patient NPO initially to protect the airway. Position the patient with the head midline and the head of bed elevated no more than 30 degrees to decrease risk of aspiration and increase cerebral perfusion. If the patient must lie flat, turn the patient on his or her side to minimize aspiration of secretions. Monitoring of vital signs, neurological status and cardiac status is also important. This is an acutely ill patient who is currently medically unstable.

7. What would you do first for this patient?

Stabilize the respiratory system. Then initiate an intravenous line for fluid balance and the administration of medications as needed; monitor vital signs and blood glucose. Place on heart monitor. In a monitored unit, vital signs, heart rhythm and oxygen saturation may be continuously monitored but do not replace nursing assessment.

Simulation 9: Sickle Cell Anemia

1. What is your interpretation of the vital signs? T 99.4°F, P 96, R 26, B/P 116/72, Pain 9/10

The pulse and blood pressure are normal. The temperature is slightly evaluated. An infection, tissue injury, and illness can cause the temperature to increase. The respiratory rate is also elevated. Any condition that results in a decrease in oxygen in the blood can cause an increase in the depth and rate of respirations. The sickling of red blood cells can cause tissue hypoxia and necrosis. As a result, the patient often experience severe pain during a sickle cell crisis.

2. Why has this patient been placed on bed rest?

Severe pain can be disabling. Bedrest is needed to help decrease metabolic requirements. Safety precautions must also be implemented when a patient receives narcotic medications.

3. Is each medication safe to administer to this patient?

All of the medications listed are common medications given to a patient with Sickle Cell Crisis.
Hydroxyurea (hydrea) 1000 mg—used to decrease painful crises and the need for transfusions in sickle cell anemia patients.
Folic Acid (folvite) 1 mg—stimulates the production of red blood cells.
Colace (docusate sodium) 100 mg—used to soften stools. Appropriate for a patient who has limited mobility and irregular eating habits.
Motrin (ibuprofen) 600 mg—used to decrease mild to moderate pain and inflammation.
Ferrous sulfate 325 mg—iron sulfate dietary supplement used to improve anemia status, hemoglobin status.
Morphine sulfate 10–15 mg—administered for moderate to severe pain. Has rapid onset but a shorter half-life than other routes. Note respiratory side effects.
Toradol (ketorolac) 15 mg—used to decrease pain.
Tylenol (acetaminophen) 650 mg po—produces analgesia and decreases body temperature. It is used to relieve mild to moderate pain and decrease fever.

4. What should you consider to determine which prn medication is appropriate for this patient?

The nurse must conduct a pain assessment. This patient has had previous hospitalizations for Sickle Cell Crisis. The patient should be asked how her pain has been managed in the past. Previous pain medications received should be reviewed and the patient should be asked how the medications previously administered worked.

5. What is your primary problem for this patient?

The priority problem for this patient is hypoxia. Priority nursing assessments must include assessment of the cardiovascular and respiratory systems. Pain is a concern; however, the pain is occurring because of decrease circulating oxygen.

6. What are your priority assessments for this patient?

The first priority assessment for this patient is oxygen. The cardiopulmonary system must be assessed closely and nursing interventions to improve oxygenation must be implemented. It is also important to conduct a pain assessment. Many patients who experience Sickle Cell Crisis have severe discomfort. Understanding the location, type, quality, intensity, duration, and aggravating and alleviating factors will help the nurse to conduct appropriate nursing interventions to manage the pain.

Simulation 10: Chronic Kidney Disease

1. What is your interpretation of the vital signs?

The admission VS were: T 100.1°F, P 98, R 20, BP142/84, SpO2 95% RA. The temperature and blood pressure are elevated. Ask the patient how long he or she has had an elevated temperature. Review labs and continue to monitor the temperature. The patient has a history of hypertension. Determine the baseline blood pressure for this patient and review the MAR to verify when she received the last dose of hypertensive medication. The pulse, respiratory rate, and oxygen saturation are WNL.

2. What is a precipitating factor that could have contributed to the development of Ms. Miles CRF?

Ms. Miles had hypertension for several years before she developed CKD. Hypertension is a common cause of CKD and CRF.

3. Why is each medication prescribed for this patient?

Lopressor (metoprolol) 100mg—Metoprolol 50 mg – a beta-blocker that reduces the heart rate, decreases the cardiac output, and lowers blood pressure. It is used to treat hypertension.

Nifedipine (Procardia) 10mg—a calcium channel blocker that dilates the blood vessels, decreases peripheral vascular resistance, decreases the workload of the heart, and improves cardiac output. It is used to treat hypertension.

Lasix (furosemide) 60mg—inhibits the reabsorption of excess fluid. It is used to decrease edema and lower blood pressure. The nurse must monitor the blood pressure and evaluate for edema. Potassium level should be monitored.

Epoetin (erythropoietin) 4000 units—stimulates the production of red blood cells. It is used to treat anemia.

Tylenol (acetaminophen) 650mg—produces analgesia and decreases body temperature. It is used to relieve mild to moderate pain and decrease fever.

4. How does renal failure affect the metabolism of medications?

As people age, they undergo normal physiological changes in kidney function. When combined with these normal physiological changes, Kidney Disease can make it difficult for the kidneys to continue functioning adequately. Older people who are required to take medication because of other medical problems are at a higher risk for further decline in kidney function. This additional lessening of kidney function can result from the kidneys experiencing an alteration in glomerular filtration, renal function, or renal clearance. Therefore, all medications must be taken with precautions.

5. What is your primary problem for this patient?

The primary problem for this patient is fluid retention. Her kidney disease has progressed to the final stage. As a result, her kidneys are unable to excrete metabolic waste and the end products of metabolism build up in the blood. Other concerns for this patient are shortness of breath and anemia.

APPENDIX B

Glossary of Terms

Alzheimer's disease—progressive mental deterioration (loss of memory, math ability, confusion) that typically begins in late middle-age; usually results in death in 5–10 years

Anorexia—lack of appetite

Arteriovenous fistula—a connection between an artery and vein that allows blood to bypassing the capillaries and flow directly from an artery to a vein

Bronchospasm—sudden constriction of the muscles in the walls of the bronchioles

Cerebral Vascular Accident—acute impairment of cerebral circulation that lasts longer than 24 hours

Chronic bronchitis—chronic inflammation of the bronchi (medium-size airways) in the lungs

Chronic Kidney Disease—a disorder that results in decrease kidney function over an extended period of time

Chronic Obstructive Pulmonary Disease—chronic bronchitis and emphysema, a pair of commonly co-existing diseases of the lungs in which the airways become narrowed

Chronic Renal Failure—a disorder in which the renal function declines slowly

Dementia—loss of cognitive and intellectual functioning. Characterized by disorientation with impaired memory and judgment

Diabetic ketoacidosis—an accumulation of ketone bodies and acidosis during the advanced stages of diabetes mellitus

Diabetes Mellitus—a metabolic disease where carbohydrate use is reduced caused by lack of insulin production or use

Diabetes Mellitus type 1—type of diabetes that commonly occurs in children or adolescents. The pancreas produces a small amount of insulin or no insulin. This results in severe insulin deficiency

Diabetes Mellitus type 2—type of diabetes that commonly occurs in adults. The insulin produced is unable to meet the body's needs

Dyspnea—the experience of unpleasant or uncomfortable respiratory sensation of shortness of breath

Edema—abnormal accumulation of fluid beneath the skin or in one or more cavities of the body

Emphysema—long-term, progressive disease of the lung that primarily causes shortness of breath

End Stage Renal Disease—the final stage of Chronic Renal Failure

Erythrocyte—mature red blood cell that contains hemoglobin and carries oxygen to the body

Gestational diabetes—hormonal changes that arise during pregnancy which causes an elevated blood glucose resulting diabetes mellitus

Heart failure—reduced pumping function of the heart. Can be right-sided, left-sided, or both

Hematochezia—fecal material with bright red blood

Hemiparesis—weakness affecting one side of the body

Hemoglobin—iron containing protein that carries oxygen from the lungs to the tissues and carbon dioxide from the tissues to the lungs

Hemolytic anemia—disorder that results in the premature destruction and removal of red blood cells

Hemorrhagic stroke—stroke caused from sudden leakage of blood into area of the brain from ruptured blood vessel

Hyperglycemia—elevated blood glucose

Hyperosmolar Hyperglycemic Nonketotic Syndrome—exceptionally high blood glucose level without the occurrence of ketones

Hypoglycemia—low blood glucose level

Hypovolemia—decreased fluid volume that occurs when the extracellular fluid volume exceeds adequate fluid intake

Hypersensitivity—any kind of unusual sensitivity or reaction

Hypothyroidism—diminished production of thyroid hormone

Hypoxia—body as a whole or region of the body is deprived of adequate oxygen supply

Infarction—deprivation of venous or arterial blood supply that result in the death of body tissue

Insulin—hormone produced in the beta cells of the pancreas that is responsible for controlling the cellular uptake of sugars, fat, protein, and metabolism

Intestinal obstruction—partial or complete blockage of the bowel

Ischemia—constriction or obstruction of a blood vessel that causes a deficiency of blood flow

Ischemic stroke—blockage of blood flow from an embolus or clot to an area of the brain

Juvenile diabetes—diabetes mellitus that develops in childhood or adolescence. Also known as type 1 diabetes

Lipoatrophy—deterioration of the subcutaneous tissue

Lipodystropy—disruption of fat metabolism

Pallor—paleness of the skin

Polydipsia—symptom in several conditions that cause's excessive thirst

Polyphagia—eating an excessive amount of food

Polyuria—increased amount of urine secretion and outflow

Mastectomy—surgical excision of the breast

Pulse oximetry—non-invasive method allowing the monitoring of the oxygenation of a patient's hemoglobin

Sickling—low oxygen tension levels that result in the production of crescent-shaped red blood cells

Sickle Cell Crisis—crescent-shaped red blood cells clumped together and impede flow in people with Sickle Cell Anemia

Sickle Cell Anemia—disease that causes the body to produce crescent-shaped red blood cells when exposed to a decrease in oxygen. The cells will become rigid, sticky, clump together and impeded blood flow

Small Bowel Obstruction—the blockage of intestinal contents in the small bowel

Transient ischemic attack—sudden focal loss of neurologic function that resolves within 24 hours; caused by brief interruption of perfusion to an area of the brain

Abbreviation List

Abbreviation	Meaning
ABG	arterial blood gas
AC	before meals
ADA Diet	American Diabetic Association Diet
ADLs	activities of daily living
Am	morning
AV	Arteriovenous
BID	two times a day
BM	bowel movement
B/P	blood pressure
BS	blood sugar
CAD	coronary artery disease
CBC	complete blood count
CXR	chest x-ray
CKD	Chronic Kidney Disease
CRF	Chronic Renal Failure
Chem	Chemistry
CHF	congestive heart failure
cm	centimeter
c/o	complaints of
Coag	coagulation
COPD	Chronic Obstructive Pulmonary Disease
CT	computed tomography
CVA	cerebral vascular accident
DKA	Diabetic Ketoacidosis
DOE	dyspnea on exertion
DM	diabetes mellitus
D_5W	Dextrose 5% in water
ED	emergency department
EKG:	electrocardiogram
ESRD	end stage renal disease
F	Fahrenheit
FeSO4	iron sulfate
HA	headache
Hb S	hemogloblin S (sickled cell hemogloblin)
HCT	hematocrit
HGB	hemoglobin
HHNS	Hyperosmolar Hyperglycemic Nonketotic Syndrome
HOB	head of bed
hr	hour
HS	bedtime
HTN	hypertension
HX	history
IDDM	insulin-dependent diabetes mellitus
IM	intramuscular
IN	inches
I/O	intake/output
IS	incentive spirometry

Abbreviation	Meaning
IV	intravenous
JP	Jackson Pratt
L	liter
lbs	pounds
LR	lactated ringers
MAR	medication administration record
max	maximum
mEq	milliequivalent
MI	myocardial infarction (heart attack)
min	minute
mg	milligram
mL	milliliter
MRI	magnetic resonance image
NaCl	sodium chloride
NC	nasal cannula
NG	nasogastric
NIDDM	non-insulin-dependent diabetes mellitus
NPO	nothing per os (mouth)
NS	normal saline
ORIF	open reduction internal fixation
OT	occupational therapy
O_2	oxygen
P	pulse
prn	as needed
po	by mouth
PT	physical therapy
q	every
QD	every day
R	respiration
RA	room air
SOB	shortness of breath
s/p	status post
SpO_2	pulse oximetry
Subcut	subcutaneous
q	every
qd	every day
q4h	every 4 hours
q6h	every 6 hours
R	temperature
RA	room air
TCDB	turn cough & deep breath
TIA	transient ischemic attack
TID	three times a day
UA	urinalysis
UAP	unlicensed assistive personnel
VS	vital signs
WNL	within normal limits
y/o	year old

NOTES

NOTES

NOTES

NOTES

NOTES

NOTES